Content Specialists

Reviewers and Contributors

Dental Health
Mary Banas
Program Specialist
Bureau of Health Education and
Audiovisual Services
American Dental Association
Chicago, Illinois

Drug Education
Chwcc Lye Chng
Assistant Professor
Division of Health Education
North Texas State University
Denton, Texas

Merita Thompson
Professor
Department of Health Education
Eastern Kentucky University
Richmond, Kentucky

Family Life Education
Linda Berne
Professor
Department of Health and Physical
Education
The University of North Carolina
Charlotte, North Carolina

Nutrition
Jean Mayer
President
Tufts University
Medford, Massachusetts

Safety and First Aid
Janice Sutkus
Technical Specialist
National Safety Council
Chicago, Illinois

Lourdes Alcorta-Rogover
Educational Consultant
Former Teacher
Miami, Florida

Ruth Ann Althaus
Professor of Public Health
Master of Public Health Program
Illinois Benedictine College
Lisle, Illinois

Matthew Bustamante
Bilingual/Cross-Cultural
Education Specialist
Bandini Elementary School
Montebello, California

Judi Coffey
Educational Consultant
Learning Disabilities Specialist
Jonesboro, Arkansas

Bryan Cooke
Professor
Department of Community Health
College of Health and Human
Services
University of Northern Colorado
Greeley, Colorado

Gail Daud
Teacher in Gifted Education
Spring Shadows Elementary School
Houston, Texas

Bo Fernhall
Director, Fitness and Cardiac
Rehabilitation
Department of Physical Education
Northern Illinois University
DeKalb, Illinois

Linda Froschauer
Teacher
Weston Public Schools
Weston, Connecticut

Rosalyn Gantt
Teacher
Midway Elementary School
Cincinnati, Ohio

Jon Hisgen
School Health Coordinator
Pewaukee Public Schools
Pewaukee, Wisconsin

Peter Loudis
Teacher of Gifted and Talented
Spring Branch Junior High School
Houston, Texas

Jeanne Mannings
Teacher
Adamsville Elementary School
Atlanta, Georgia

Wanda Nottingham-Brooks
Learning Disabilities Teacher
Morrisonville Junior and Senior
High School
Morrisonville, Illinois

Bert Pearlman
Director, Curriculum Research
and Evaluation
Office of the County
Superintendent of Schools
Santa Barbara, California

Candace Purdy
Health Teacher
Maine South High School
Park Ridge, Illinois

Joan Salmon
School Nurse
Greenwood School Corporation
Greenwood, Indiana

David R. Stronck
Associate Professor of Health
Education
Department of Teacher Education
California State University, Hayward
Hayward, California

Shirley Van Sickle
Health Teacher
DeVeaux Junior High School
Toledo, Ohio

Chapter 1   You and Your Feelings 16

Chapter 2

Food and Your Health 38

Chapter 3   You and Your Body 66

Chapter 4

Caring For Your Teeth 92

Chapter 5   You and Your Safety   120

Chapter 7   Your Physical Fitness   172

Chapter 8   A Healthy Community   198

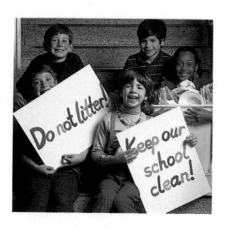

Why Learn About Health

"When you have your health, you have just about everything." You might have heard this saying before. What does it mean to you? Most people agree that good health is one of the most important things a person could have. When you are healthy, you can enjoy life more fully. Good health helps you think clearly and get along with others at school. Good health keeps your body working properly so you can enjoy your play. Good health helps you look and feel your best.

Learning about health is important because you are making more and more decisions about your own health. For example, you might decide what to eat for lunch or where to play after school.

To make the wisest decisions, you need good information. Then you need to know how to use this information. Finally, you need to develop *skills for life.* These skills will help you deal with events in your life in good and healthful ways. Scott, Foresman's *Health for Life* gives you the tools that can improve your health, but it is up to you to use them. Make good health a part of your day and a part of your life, now and in the years to come.

When You Read This Book

1. Read the question.

1 | **Who Is Most Responsible for Keeping You Safe?**

Suppose you were waiting to cross the street as this girl is doing. What would you do before crossing? What is the safe way to be sure you cross after all cars have stopped?

The girl knows that she is responsible for keeping herself safe. She is following a safety rule that she has learned. She always waits on the curb and looks left, right, and then left again before crossing any street. Following this rule helps keep her safe.

Just like this girl, you are responsible for keeping yourself safe. Other people can only help keep you safe. You are most responsible for your own safety. Following safety rules can help keep you safe.

3. Find the answer.

This girl looks to the left, right, and then left again to keep herself safe.

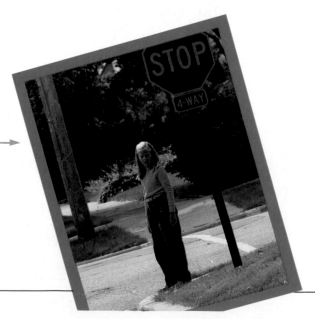

2. Look at the pictures.

4. Learn the health word.

Being careful can help keep you safe. For example, you can help prevent an **injury** when you watch where you walk on stairs. You do not want to fall and hurt yourself. Hold on to a railing if possible.

injury (in′jər ē), damage to the body.

Thinking of ways to prevent accidents can also help keep you safe. Suppose you and your friends want to play ball in the park. Before you play, you should carefully check the playing field for sharp objects. How might this rule help prevent injuries?

Think back • *Study on your own with Study Guide page 230.*

1. Who is most responsible for your safety?
2. What can help a person be a safe walker?
3. What can a person do to help prevent accidents?

5. Use what you learned.

You and Your Feelings

What different feelings does this girl have? You have different feelings too. This chapter will tell you about the different feelings that people have. Knowing about different feelings can help you get along with others now and in the future.

Health Watch Notebook

Collect pictures of your friends or the people in your family. Under each picture, write a sentence about what helps you get along with that person.

feelings, the way a person feels about something.

On Your Own
Each child in the picture feels differently about the rainstorm that spoiled their picnic. Write a paragraph explaining why each child feels as he or she does.

1 How Do You and Others Show Feelings?

Sometimes you might feel happy or sad or angry. Sometimes you might feel worried or disappointed or surprised. Happiness, sadness, anger, worry, and surprise are **feelings.** You have feelings and so does everyone else.

Sometimes faces show how people feel. Look at the children's faces shown here. It rained just as they were going on a picnic. How do you think each child feels about the rainstorm?

Sometimes voices show how people feel. Bill said in an angry voice, "Why did it rain and spoil our picnic?" Can you make your voice sound angry like Bill's voice?

Sometimes people show feelings in the way they stand or move. Look again at the children in the pictures. Does the way each is standing help show his or her feelings? How might someone who feels proud walk?

Think Back • *Study on your own with Study Guide page 222.*

1. What are some feelings people have?
2. What are some ways people show their feelings?

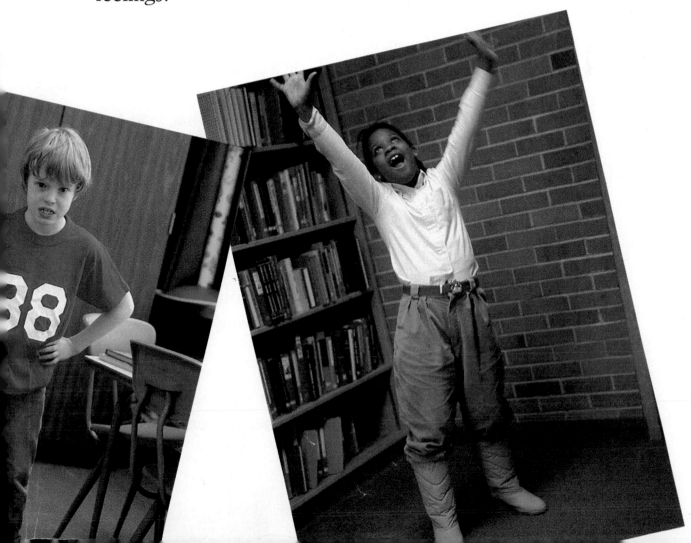

2 What Can Help When You Feel Scared?

Jenny and some friends planned a play. Jenny is to play the part of a space traveler. She feels scared on the day of the play. Jenny wants to be in the play. At the same time, she does not want to be in the play. What can help Jenny's scared feelings?

Everyone feels scared at certain times. Remembering this might help you feel better when you are scared. You might have scared feelings when you start to learn new things. You might have scared feelings because you are afraid of not doing something well.

Sometimes talking about scared feelings helps you feel better. Talking with a family member, a friend, or a teacher might help you feel less scared.

Many times it helps to do what you feel scared about doing. Then your scared feelings might soon go away. You might not think about being scared if you are doing something. What is Jenny doing to help herself feel less scared?

Can you think of times when people might feel scared? What could help make their scared feelings go away?

Think Back • *Study on your own with Study Guide page 222.*

1. When might a person feel scared?
2. What might help when a person has scared feelings?

3 What Can Help When Feelings Are Hurt?

Glen laughed when Melissa made a mistake. Glen did not mean to hurt Melissa's feelings, but he did. Now Glen is feeling sad and worried. He knows he did an unkind thing. He thinks Melissa might not play with him anymore. What can Glen do to make things better?

You might want to talk to a family member if you have hurt someone's feelings. You might also talk to a friend. Ask for advice about how you can make the person whose feelings you hurt feel better.

Saying "I'm sorry" can help change hurt feelings.

Often saying two words can help change hurt feelings. The words are "I'm sorry." In the picture, Glen is saying these words to his friend Melissa. How can saying "I'm sorry" help?

Suppose a person often says or does unkind things to others. Then, saying the words "I'm sorry" might not help change hurt feelings. The person must act differently so that he or she does not hurt the feelings of others.

On Your Own
The boy in the picture is saying "I'm sorry" to his friend. List on paper three other things he can do to help change his friend's hurt feelings.

Think Back • *Study on your own with Study Guide page 222.*

1. Who might give advice about how to make a person with hurt feelings feel better?
2. What two words can be said to help change hurt feelings?

4 What Can Help When a Pet Dies?

Danny had a dog named Sparky. Danny loved Sparky very much. Danny had his pet for six years. One day a car hit Sparky and the pet died. Danny felt very sad. What is Danny doing to help himself feel better?

Talking to family members might help a person whose pet has died. Family members often know that the person feels very sad. Family members might suggest ways to help the person feel better.

You might like to know how Danny's family helped him. What did different family members say to Danny?

Danny's grandfather said, "You go ahead and cry. Crying often helps a sad person feel better."

Danny's mother said, "You can always remember Sparky. Think of what you and Sparky liked to do together."

Danny's younger sister said, "I will draw a picture of Sparky for you. Then you can remember how Sparky looked."

What are some other ways family members might help a sad person feel better?

Talking to family members can help when a person feels sad.

Think Back • *Study on your own with Study Guide page 223.*

1. How might talking to family members help a person whose pet has died?
2. What can a person whose pet has died do to feel better?

5 What Can Help When Things Go Wrong?

Suppose you have a day when things go wrong. You are late for school. You lose your spelling paper. Two friends go off to play without you after school. How might you feel?

You might feel angry and upset when things go wrong. What could you do to help change these feelings?

You might try doing something active. Exercising can often help you feel better. You might go outdoors to play. You might toss a ball or run for a while.

You might do something you think you will enjoy. Doing something enjoyable can help you feel better when you feel angry and upset. What are these children enjoying doing?

You might do something for others to help yourself feel better. Maybe you can help at home in some way. Ask an adult in your family what you can do to help. You often feel better when you are busy. You might start to feel less angry and upset.

Think Back • *Study on your own with Study Guide page 223.*

1. How might a person feel when things go wrong?
2. What can a person do to help change angry and upset feelings?

Doing something enjoyable can sometimes help a person feel better.

Learning More About Feelings

1. Look at the puzzle. Read from left to right. Find the names of seven feelings all people have. Write the names on your own paper.

```
Z V N M S A D X X O P W
H A P P Y V X A N G R Y
Y R E S C A R E D X V C
O H U R T E W Q Q A Z X
E E P R O U D C C B N Y
V E T W W O R R I E D O
```

2. Make up a play about how family members can help a person whose pet has died. Ask your classmates to play the parts of family members.

3. This boy is drawing an activity that he enjoys doing. What activities do you enjoy doing? Draw yourself doing them. Keep your drawings. Look at them when you are feeling angry and upset. Choose one of the activities to do to help you feel better.

4. Do you like to draw pictures? You might want to be an **artist** if you do. Some artists go to a special art school. They learn to do different kinds of art, including drawing and painting.

Artists show their feelings through their work. People who look at works of art can have different feelings about them.

Some artists sell their artwork. Some artists teach art classes. Some artists draw pictures for books. Artists might also work for companies. The artists help make up advertisements for the companies. The advertisements are put on television or in newspapers and magazines.

Look at this painting. What feelings do you think the artist is trying to show? What feelings might a person have when looking at the painting?

You might like to find a book of paintings in a library. Think of the different feelings the paintings show.

sharing, using something together.

cooperation
(kō op′ə rā′shən), working together with other people.

6 What Can Help You Get Along with Others?

Amy is feeling troubled and a little puzzled too. She has just had an argument with her younger brother. Each one wanted to use the same tube of glue. Amy and her brother argued about who would use the glue first. Amy sometimes asks herself, "Do all sisters and brothers have arguments?" How would you answer Amy's question?

People who love each other, such as people in a family, might argue at times. All sisters and brothers argue a little. However, too much arguing can upset people.

Why might sisters and brothers argue? Often they argue about taking turns or **sharing** games and toys. Sharing means using things together or dividing things up and each getting a part.

People in families can argue less if they learn to share. Sharing can also help you get along with others. How are Amy and her brother sharing here?

You also get along better with others if you work together to get jobs done. You show **cooperation** when you do your best to work with other people. Family members might show cooperation when doing jobs around the house. How could you show cooperation in other ways at home?

Sharing helps people
get along better.

consideration
(kən sid′ə rā′shən),
thinking about another
person's feelings.

On Your Own
Make a list of ways you
can show consideration
for a new person. Try to
list at least three ways.
Use the ways if a new
person comes to your
classroom.

How Can Showing Consideration Help?

These children are asking a new student at their school to play with them. They know that a new person often feels lonely. They want the newcomer to feel happy. They are showing **consideration** for the new person.

Suppose you see a new person at school. The new person looks sad and lonely. He or she cannot hear well. You could show consideration by asking the person to choose a game to play. The newcomer might choose a game in which hearing well is not important.

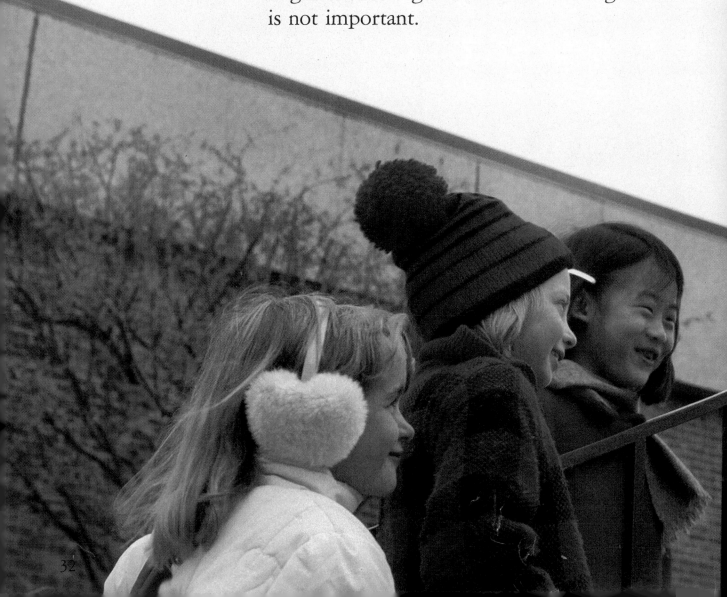

32

How Can Showing Understanding Help?

Showing **understanding** for someone who makes a mistake can help the person feel better. You show understanding when you try to think of how another person feels. You might say this to a person who makes a mistake: "Try not to feel bad. You're not the only one who ever makes mistakes."

understanding, knowing what another person is feeling.

Think Back • *Study on your own with Study Guide page 223.*

1. How can sharing help people?
2. How can showing consideration for a new person help him or her?
3. How can you show understanding when someone makes a mistake?

Vikki Carr Sings Away Her Shyness

Vikki Carr is a famous singer who sings in concerts and on television. She has even sung at the White House for two United States Presidents. She sings in English and in Spanish. Many people enjoy listening to her.

Vikki Carr has always enjoyed singing. However, as a young girl she was shy. Her teachers did not think she would go into show business because of her shyness. Vikki Carr had to get over her shy feelings to be a singer. She went on stage even though she felt shy. She got over being shy after singing in front of people many times.

Look at the picture of Vikki Carr singing. What do you think she is feeling? How would you feel if you were singing in front of many people? Vikki Carr is proud to sing on stage.

Talk About It

1. How did Vikki Carr get over her shy feelings?
2. What could feeling less shy help a person do?

Vikki Carr singing the National Anthem at a political convention

Having Happy Feelings

Do you like it when people at home have happy feelings? You can make even more of those happy feelings. You might do this activity.

Each week, find something kind or helpful to do for people in your family. Do not tell what you will do. Just go ahead and be kind or helpful. Then wait to see what happens.

What is this girl doing? How might she make a person feel happy? What could you do at home to be kind or helpful?

Reading at Home

Every Kids Guide to Coping with Childhood Traumas by Joy Berry. Childrens Press, 1988. Learn steps to help you deal with painful experiences.

Health and Friends by Dorothy Baldwin. Rourke, 1987. Discover what makes friendships work.

Chapter 1 Review

Reviewing Lesson Objectives
1. Tell ways people can show feelings. (pages 18–19)
2. Tell what can help when a person has scared feelings. (pages 20–21)
3. Tell what two words can be said to help change hurt feelings. (pages 22–23)
4. Tell what a person whose pet has died can do to feel better. (pages 24–25)
5. Tell what a person can do to help change angry and upset feelings. (pages 26–27)
6. Tell how sharing and showing cooperation, consideration, and understanding help a person. (pages 30–33)

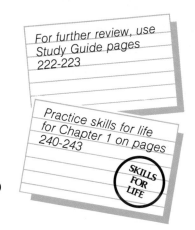

For further review, use Study Guide pages 222-223

Practice skills for life for Chapter 1 on pages 240-243

SKILLS FOR LIFE

Checking Health Vocabulary
Number your paper from 1–5. Match each meaning in Column I with the correct word in Column II.

Column I
1. the way a person feels about something
2. using something together
3. working together with other people
4. thinking about another person's feelings
5. knowing what another person is feeling

Column II
a. consideration
b. cooperation
c. feelings
d. sharing
e. understanding

Number your paper from 6–9. Next to each number write the word that best completes each sentence in the paragraph. Choose the words from the list below.

enjoys   exercising   others   upset

A person might feel __(6)__ when things go wrong. Sometimes __(7)__ can help the person feel better. Doing something he or she __(8)__ can help too. Often doing something for __(9)__ helps a person feel better.

36

Reviewing Health Ideas

Number your paper from 1–8. Next to each number write the word that best completes the sentence. Choose the words from the list below.

faces scared
family share
hurt stand
others understanding

1. Sometimes people's _____ show their feelings.
2. Sometimes people show feelings in the way they _____ or move.
3. Many times _____ feelings go away if a person goes ahead and does something.
4. Often saying "I'm sorry" can change _____ feelings.
5. Talking to _____ members might help a person whose pet has died.
6. Doing something for _____ might help a person feel less angry and upset.
7. People in families might argue less if they learn to _____ .
8. Showing _____ for someone who makes a mistake can help the person feel better.

Understanding Health Ideas

Number your paper from 9–15. Next to each number write the word or words that best answer the question.

9. What are happiness, anger, disappointment, and surprise?
10. What might a scared person remember to feel less scared?
11. What should a person do if he or she often hurts others' feelings?
12. How might crying help a sad person?
13. What is an activity that a person might do to feel less angry or upset?
14. How might family members show cooperation at home?
15. What might people show for a newcomer to help them feel happy?

Thinking Critically

Write the answers on your paper. Use complete sentences.

1. What are some ways you might show cooperation at school?
2. What are some ways you might show understanding for your classmates?

37

2

Food and Your Health

Only healthy foods are being used to make these muffins. What foods would you choose to make a healthy snack?

This chapter will teach you to make healthy food choices. You will learn healthy ways to prepare food. Knowing how to choose, prepare, and serve healthy food can help you throughout your life.

Health Watch Notebook

Collect pictures or ads of healthy foods and put them in your notebook. Write which food group each food belongs to.

nutrient (nü′trē ənt), a substance from food that is needed for health and growth.

1 What Can Help You Make Healthy Food Choices?

A grocery store has many different kinds of foods to choose from. Most of the foods are in attractive packages. People often have a difficult time deciding which foods to buy. Think of the reasons why you choose the foods you do. You might choose foods because you like their taste, smell, or color.

Eric and his mother are shopping for groceries. How can Eric's mother decide which foods her family needs?

Eric's mother uses the four food group plan to help her choose healthy foods. Your family and you can use this plan too. The plan tells what four main kinds of foods you need every day. The plan also tells how much of each kind of food to eat.

Eric and his mother are using the four food group plan to make healthy food choices.

40

Using the plan helps you get the right **nutrients.** Foods have nutrients your body needs. Some nutrients give you energy. Other nutrients help your body grow. Still other nutrients help your body work as it should.

You cannot get all the nutrients your body needs from just one kind of food. You need to eat different kinds of food each day. The nutrients in different kinds of food work together to help you stay healthy.

Pages 42 and 43 show the four food groups and explain the plan. Study the plan to answer these questions.

- What are the four food groups?
- What are some foods in each group?
- How many servings of food from each group do you need every day?

vegetable-fruit group, the food group that has vegetables and fruits.

bread-cereal group, the food group that has grains and foods made from grains.

What Are the Four Food Groups?

The pictures show the four food groups. Find out how each group can help your body. One food group has grains and foods made from grains. What is the name of this group? What foods are in the same group as meat?

Vegetable-fruit group

Most of the nutrients in these foods help your body work as it should. You need four servings from the **vegetable-fruit group** each day.

Bread-cereal group

Most of the nutrients in these foods give your body energy. You need four servings from the **bread-cereal group** each day.

Think Back • *Study on your own with Study Guide page 224.*

1. What can be used to help make healthy food choices?
2. How do nutrients help keep the body healthy?
3. What are the names of the four food groups?
4. How many servings from each food group are needed each day?

meat-poultry-fish-bean group, the food group that has meats, poultry, fish, nuts, eggs, and beans.

milk-cheese group, the food group that has milk and foods made from milk.

Meat-poultry-fish-bean group

Milk-cheese group

Most of the nutrients in these foods help your body grow. You need two servings from the **meat-poultry-fish-bean group** each day.

The foods in this group have many different kinds of nutrients. Some nutrients help your body grow. Some nutrients give you energy. Some help your body work as it should. You need three servings from the **milk-cheese group** each day.

2 What Are Some Healthy Meals?

Look at what Jill ate one day for breakfast, lunch, and supper. Did she eat healthy meals?

Jill ate foods from each of the four food groups. Healthy meals for a day have foods from each food group. Jill had orange juice, vegetable soup, an apple, and salad from the vegetable-fruit group. She had oatmeal, toast, rice, and a roll from the bread-cereal group. She had peanut butter and chicken from the meat group. From the milk-cheese group she had yogurt and two glasses of milk.

Healthy meals for a day have enough servings from each food group. Jill had enough servings from each group. She ate four servings from the vegetable-fruit group. She ate four servings from the bread-cereal group. She ate two servings from the meat group and three servings from the milk-cheese group.

Suppose you were planning Jill's meals for tomorrow. What foods would your menu have to give Jill energy? What foods on the menu would help her body grow? What foods would help Jill's body work as it should?

Healthy meals for a day

Breakfast

Lunch

How Can You Decide If a Day's Meals Are Healthy?

Be a food detective. Look at the meals Mike ate one day. Decide if Mike had healthy meals. Use the four food group plan to help you decide.

First, find out if Mike had foods from each of the four food groups. Look back at pages 42 and 43 if you need help.

Now, find out if Mike had enough servings from each food group. Make a chart like this one to help you decide.

What did you find out about Mike's meals?

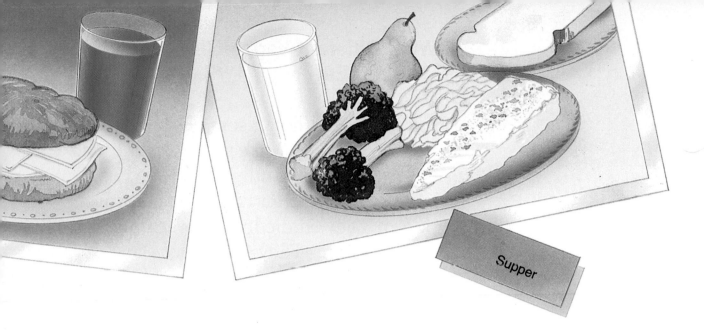

Supper

	Breakfast	Lunch	Supper	Total servings
Vegetable-fruit group 4 servings				4
Bread-cereal group 4 servings				
Meat-poultry-fish-bean group 2 servings				
Milk-cheese group 3 servings				

Think Back • *Study on your own with Study Guide page 224.*

1. How can the four food group plan be used to have healthy meals for a day?
2. What are some foods that can make up a healthy breakfast?
3. What are some foods that can make up a healthy lunch?
4. What are some foods that can make up a healthy supper?

3 What Different Vegetables Can You Eat?

Eat these kinds of vegetables three or four times weekly.

You have been doing some detective work. You checked Mike's meals and found that he was eating healthy meals.

Some other children did some detective work too. They studied what vegetables they were eating. They found out they were eating many different vegetables.

You need to eat different kinds of vegetables. Different kinds of vegetables give you different kinds of nutrients. Your body needs these nutrients to stay healthy.

All of the vegetables you eat come from parts of plants. For example, you are eating the leaves of a plant when you eat spinach. A carrot is the root of a plant.

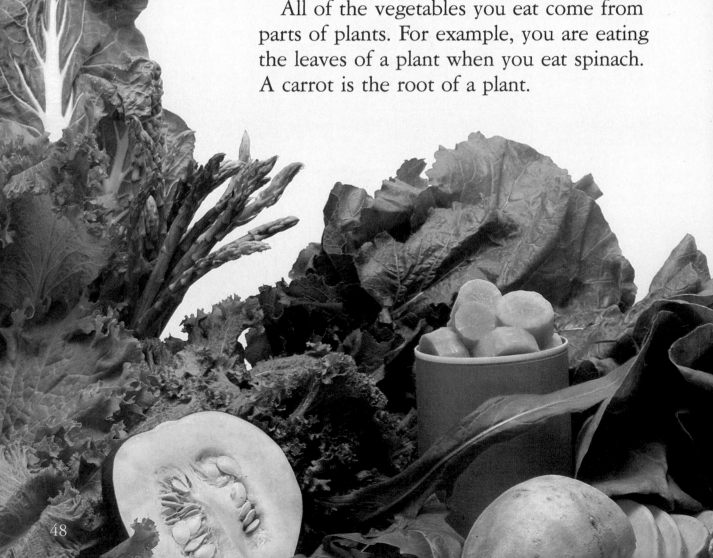

Try to eat leafy, green, or dark yellow vegetables three or four times a week. What green vegetables do you see in the picture? Which green vegetables are leafy? What dark yellow vegetables do you see?

Which vegetables do you like? Why do you like them? Do you like their colors? What special way do you like them served?

Look again at the vegetables. Which are fresh? What other ways can you see to buy vegetables?

Think Back • *Study on your own with Study Guide page 224.*

1. What kinds of vegetables should be eaten three or four times a week?
2. How can eating different kinds of vegetables help keep the body healthy?

On Your Own

Frank is eating lunch at a friend's home. Frank has never tasted the green vegetable that his friend is eating. Frank is trying to decide if he should eat the vegetable or not. What do you think Frank should do? Write a paragraph explaining why you think as you do.

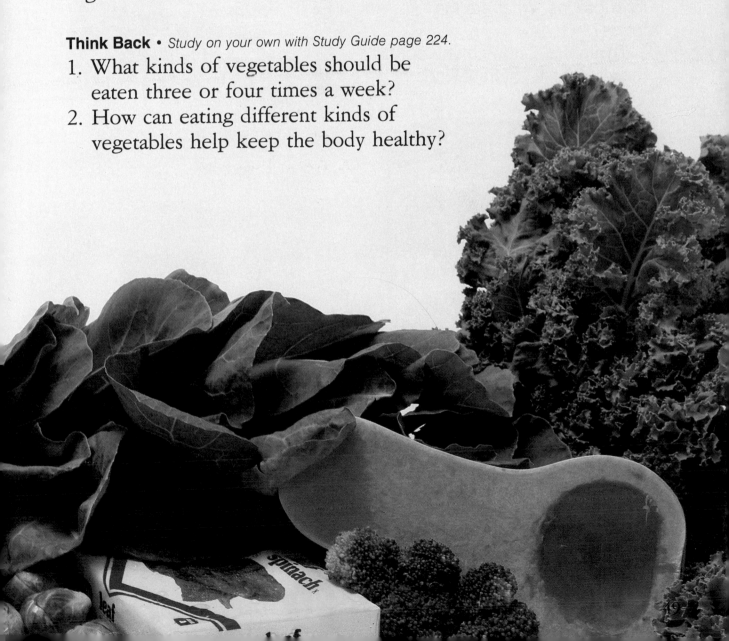

49

Learning More About Healthy Foods

1. Look at the sandwich. It has foods in it from each of the four food groups. What are the foods?

Think of a sandwich you could make. List the different kinds of food in your sandwich. Try to have a food from each food group in it.

2. Guess the answer to this riddle.

This food is in the vegetable-fruit group.

You can eat it raw or cooked.

It is a red color.

Its name starts with T.

What is it?

3. Think of a vegetable you like. Write a few sentences about it. Tell why you like the vegetable. Get an idea from what one boy wrote about why he likes corn.

You might draw a picture to go with your story.

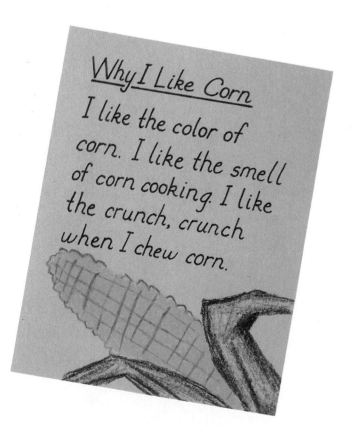

Why I Like Corn

I like the color of corn. I like the smell of corn cooking. I like the crunch, crunch when I chew corn.

▶▶ **Looking at Careers**

4. A **dietitian** plans meals for schools, hospitals, nursing homes, and some restaurants. He or she tries to make the meals as healthy as possible. A dietitian might also teach people how to plan more healthy meals. Would you enjoy this job? You need to go to college for four years to be a dietitian.

Maybe you know a dietitian. Ask the person to tell you about his or her work. You also might look for a book that tells what a dietitian does. Ask a librarian to help you.

4 How Can You Make Healthy Snack Choices?

For Joe's birthday, his mother is bringing some healthy snacks to school. The snacks are not too sweet or salty.

Sweet snacks, such as cake and candy, are not very healthy. These snacks can stick to your teeth and harm them. Try not to choose too many sweet, sticky snacks.

Fatty snacks, such as fried foods, are not healthy. These snacks can harm your heart. Try to choose snacks that are low in fat. Snacks such as low-fat milk and low-fat yogurt can help keep your heart healthy.

Try not to eat too many salty snacks. Healthy snacks have little salt added to them. Many foods from the four food groups have salt in them. You get enough salt from these foods in your meals. You do not need to add more.

Choosing healthy snacks can help you get food you need each day. Suppose you do not get enough servings of fruits and vegetables in your meals. What snacks could you choose to make up the servings?

Joe is getting ready to serve some healthy snacks at his birthday party.

What Are Some Healthy Snacks?

You can see the healthy snacks Joe's mother brought to school. What food groups are they from?

You could make some changes and still have healthy snacks. You might have green pepper slices instead of celery. What other fruit drinks might you have?.

Think Back • *Study on your own with Study Guide 225.*

1. What should a person think about when choosing healthy snacks?
2. How can eating healthy snacks help you get food you need each day?
3. What are some healthy snacks from the four food groups?

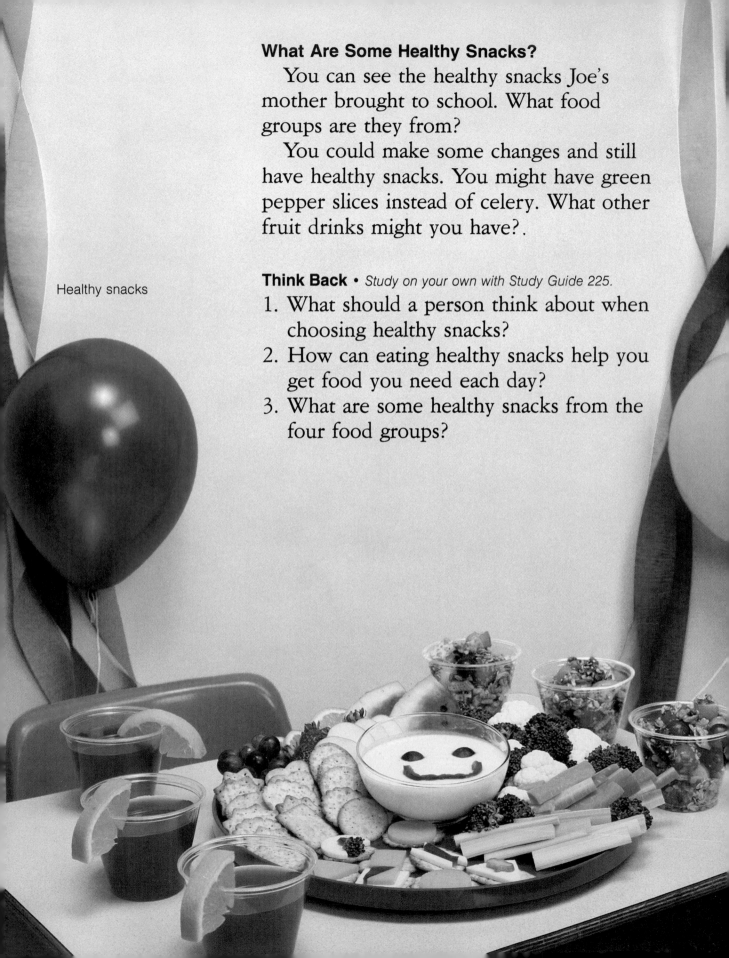

Healthy snacks

Learning More About Healthy Snacks

1. Look at the different ways to serve peanut butter. Draw pictures of some different ways to serve eggs, carrots, tomatoes, or potatoes. The pictures show some ways to serve these foods.

2. Go to a library and find a cookbook for children. Use the cookbook to help you plan a healthy snack. Ask a parent for permission to make the snack at home.

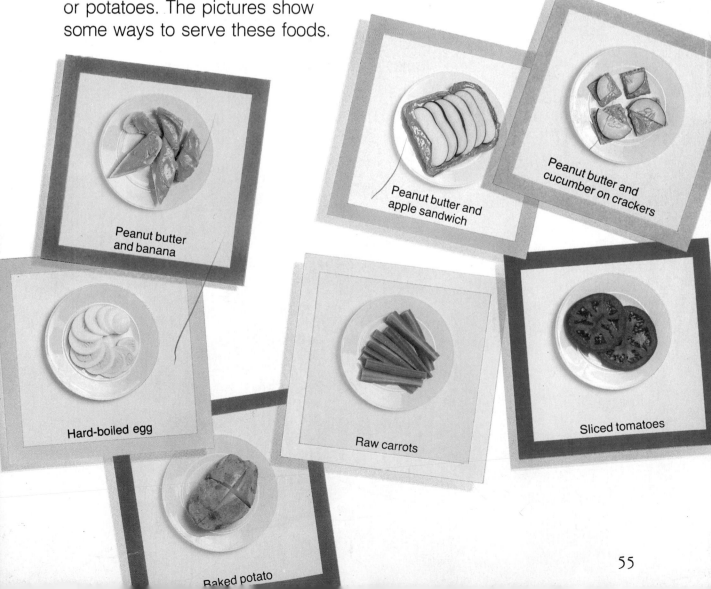

Peanut butter and apple sandwich

Peanut butter and cucumber on crackers

Peanut butter and banana

Hard-boiled egg

Raw carrots

Sliced tomatoes

Baked potato

5 How Can You Be a Wise Food Shopper?

Maria's father asked her to buy a can of fruit juice for breakfast. He said, "Buy a large can of fruit juice. Be sure you get real fruit juice." Maria wants to be a wise food shopper. What should she do?

Maria should read the labels on the cans. The labels can tell Maria what she needs to know. For example, a label can tell if a can has all real fruit juice in it. Some drinks have only flavor, water, and sugar in them. Notice the labels on the cans. Which can has all real fruit juice in it?

Maria should also look at the prices of the cans. Then she can find out which kind of fruit juice will cost the least.

The label tells what is inside a can.

THIRSTY AID
CONTAINS NO FRUIT JUICE

FRUIT COOLER
10% fruit juice

Maria should be willing to try different kinds of foods. For example, she could try the kind of fruit juice that costs the least. The best tasting foods do not always cost the most. You can often find good tasting foods at lower prices. How do you find out if these foods taste good? Be willing to try them.

Suppose the kind of food that costs the least does not taste good. The wise food shopper will not buy that kind again.

Think Back • *Study on your own with Study Guide page 225.*

1. What can a wise food shopper learn from reading labels?
2. What can a wise food shopper learn from looking at prices?
3. What can a wise food shopper learn from trying different kinds of foods?

57

Learning More About Food Choices

1. Make up a play. Pretend you are in a food store with a friend. The friend wants to buy a can of baked beans. What can you tell your friend about making wise food choices?

2. Write a short story about choosing a new food for your family. Be sure to tell what the food is. You might also write why you would choose it. Do you think your story shows you made a wise food choice? Explain your answer.

3. Sometimes stores have food sales. Some foods will cost less than usual. The stores have signs like these that tell about their food sales. Make up a sign for a food sale. Tell how your sign could help a food shopper.

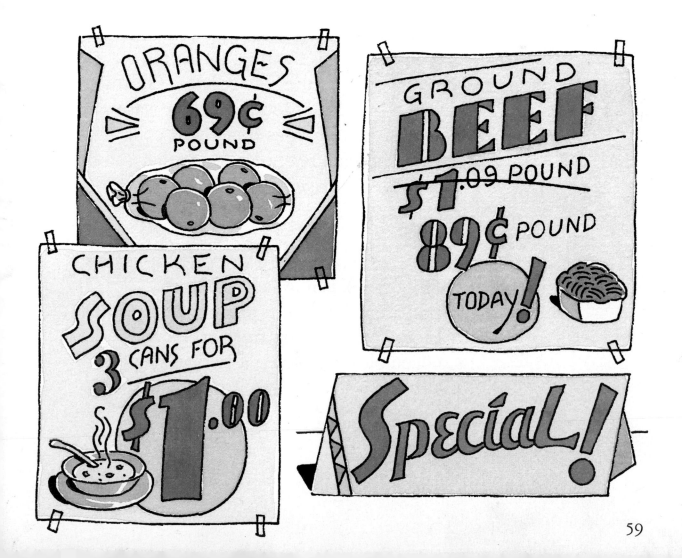

6 What Are Healthy Ways to Prepare and Serve Food?

Suppose you are going to help make supper. What should you do first?

You should wash your hands with soap and warm water. You will wash away germs that can cause disease. Germs will not get on foods you touch if your hands are clean.

Wash any fresh fruits and vegetables too. You will wash away harmful germs and chemicals when you wash them. You will also wash off dirt.

Be sure you use clean pans, dishes, and spoons. Wash the tabletop you work on as well. Why should you do this?

When you finish eating, put some leftover foods in the refrigerator. Germs can grow in certain foods that get warm. Germs do not grow as quickly in cold places. The picture shows foods that should be kept in a refrigerator. What leftover foods do you see?

Think Back • *Study on your own with Study Guide page 225.*

1. How can washing hands before preparing food help prevent disease?
2. How does washing fresh fruits and vegetables help keep a person healthy?
3. What is a healthy way to store leftover foods?

These foods
should be kept in
a refrigerator.

Making Milk Safe to Drink

Is milk one of your favorite drinks? Then you might want to say thank you to Louis Pasteur. His studies helped make milk safe for you to drink.

Louis Pasteur was born in France in 1822. As a child, he was interested in learning about science. Pasteur became a science teacher when he grew up.

One of Louis Pasteur's special interests was studying germs. He learned that some germs can cause disease. He also discovered that harmful germs die when they are heated to a certain temperature.

Later scientists learned that harmful germs were in some milk. Some people got sick after they drank milk. Some of these people died.

After many years, Pasteur's discovery about heating germs was used to kill germs in milk. This way of making milk safe to drink is named for Louis Pasteur. It is known as pasteurization. All dairies in the United States now pasteurize milk.

Talk About It
1. How did Louis Pasteur's studies help make milk safe to drink?
2. What are some other foods that are safe to eat because of Louis Pasteur's studies?

Planning Healthy Snacks with Your Family

You have learned what healthy snacks are. What can you tell your family about such snacks?

You could make plans with your family for a snack spot in your refrigerator. The picture shows some snacks you might want to put in your snack spot.

Family members might take turns preparing the snacks. Decide on times to eat the snacks.

Reading at Home

Eat Up, Gemma by Sarah Hayes. Lothrop, 1988. Baby Gemma refuses to eat anything her family offers her until her brother gets an idea that changes her mind.

Nutrition by Leslie Jean LeMaster. Children's Press, 1985. Find out how our bodies use nutrients and how poor nutrition can cause disease.

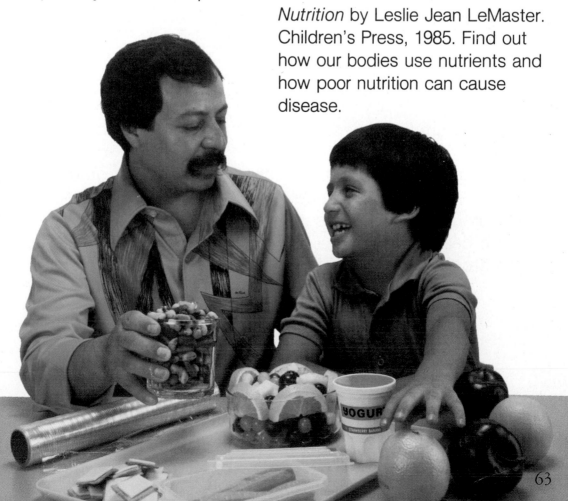

Chapter 2 Review

Reviewing Lesson Objectives

1. Tell the number of daily servings needed from each food group. (pages 40–43)
2. Tell how using the food group plan helps in planning healthy meals for a day. (pages 44–47)
3. Tell what kinds of vegetables should be eaten three or four times a week. (pages 48–49)
4. Tell what to think about when choosing healthy snacks and list some healthy snacks. (pages 52–54)
5. Tell how to be a wise food shopper. (pages 56–57)
6. Tell healthy ways to prepare, serve, and keep foods. (pages 60–61)

For further review, use Study Guide pages 224-225

Practice skills for life for Chapter 2 on pages 244-246

SKILLS FOR LIFE

Checking Health Vocabulary

Number your paper from 1–5. Match each meaning in Column I with the correct word or words in Column II.

Column I

1. a substance from food needed for health and growth
2. the food group with foods made from grain
3. the food group made up of vegetables and fruits
4. the food group that has meats, poultry, fish, nuts, eggs, and beans
5. the food group with milk and foods made from milk

Column II

a. bread-cereal group
b. meat-poultry-fish-bean group
c. milk-cheese group
d. nutrient
e. vegetable-fruit group

Reviewing Health Ideas

Number your paper from 1–8. Next to each number write the word that best completes the sentence. Choose the words from the list below.

four	nutrients
germs	snacks
labels	three
meals	vegetables

1. Food has _____ the body needs.
2. The number of servings needed each day from the milk-cheese group is _____.
3. The number of servings needed each day from the vegetable-fruit group is _____.
4. Healthy _____ for a day have foods from four food groups.
5. Leafy, green, or dark yellow _____ should be eaten three or four times a week.
6. Eating fruits for _____ can help make up needed daily servings.
7. Reading _____ helps a wise food shopper find out what is in food.
8. Washing fresh fruits and vegetables removes harmful _____ and chemicals.

Understanding Health Ideas

Number your paper from 9–15. Next to each number write the word or words that best answer the question.

9. How many daily servings are needed from the bread-cereal group?
10. How many daily servings are needed from the meat-poultry-fish-bean group?
11. What can be used to help plan healthy meals for the day?
12. What do vegetables contain to help keep the body healthy?
13. What kinds of snacks can harm the teeth?
14. What can a food shopper do to find out if a food tastes good?
15. Why are some leftover foods kept in a refrigerator?

Thinking Critically

Write the answers on your paper. Use complete sentences.

1. How does your favorite snack help you stay healthy?
2. How can trying new foods help you stay healthy?

3

You and Your Body

This sister is helping her brother find out how much he has grown in the last year. What makes his body grow?

This chapter will help you find out how your body grows and works. You might be able to take better care of your body if you understand how it works. Taking good care of your body can help keep you healthy now and in the future.

Health Watch Notebook

At the end of each day, think about how certain parts of your body helped you do something. Write a paragraph in your notebook about your thoughts.

1   What Are You Made Of?
2   How Do Your Muscles and Bones Help You?
3   How Do Your Brain and Nerves Help You?
4   How Does Your Heart Help You?
5   How Do Your Lungs Help You?
6   How Do Your Stomach and Intestines Help You?
7   How Does Your Body Grow?

1 What Are You Made Of?

The outside of you is made up of skin, hair, and nails. Inside you are such things as bones, muscles, nerves, and blood.

Every part of you is made up of very tiny living parts. Each tiny part is a **cell**. You are made of millions of cells.

Your body is made of many different kinds of cells. Each kind is a different size and shape. Each kind does a different job.

You need a microscope to see body cells.

Microscope

Bone tissue

When many cells of the same kind are grouped together, they make up **tissue**. For example, many bone cells together make up bone tissue. Many muscle cells together make up muscle tissue. Many nerve cells together make up nerve tissue.

Suppose you could look at different tissues through a microscope. You would see cells like these. Do the cells all look alike?

tissue (tish′ü), a group of cells that look alike.

Think Back • *Study on your own with Study Guide page 226.*

1. What are the smallest living parts of the body?
2. What makes up tissue?
3. What is needed to see body cells?

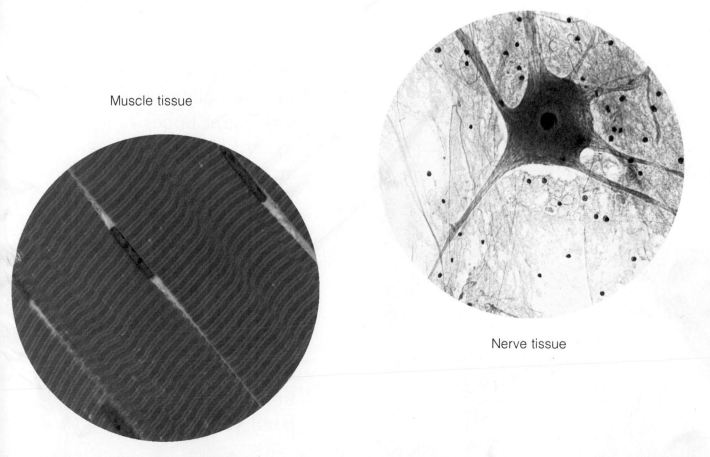

Muscle tissue

Nerve tissue

2 How Do Your Muscles and Bones Help You?

Look at the picture. It shows where muscles are in the body. Where can you find long muscles and short muscles? Where can you find flat ones?

Muscles give your body shape. Muscles also help you move about. Muscles are attached to your bones. The muscles pull the bones. The pulling makes the bones move.

Bend an arm. A muscle pulls your lower arm bones toward your upper arm bone. Straighten your arm. Another muscle pulls the lower arm bones away from the upper bone. The muscles in your body work in pairs to let you bend. Now feel the inside of your upper arm while you bend your arm.

Some muscles in the human body

Straighten your arm. Can you feel your muscles working to move your arm?

Your bones are under your muscles. You have more than two hundred bones in your body. All your bones together make up your skeleton.

Your bones help hold you up. Your bones and muscles help you move about. Your bones help give your body its shape. Some of your bones help protect parts of your body.

Notice the different kinds of bones in the skeleton. Some bones are long and some are short. Some bones are flat and some are round. Each bone has a special job to do.

Can you feel the bones in your head? What do they protect inside your head?

Bones in the human body

How Do Your Joints Help You?

Joints are the places in the skeleton where the bones fit together. Different joints let you move in different ways. The picture shows a joint in the body. You can kick a ball because of your knee joint. It lets you move your leg back and forth. Your shoulder joint lets you swing a bat. It lets you move your arm back and forth and around and around.

Think Back • *Study on your own with Study Guide page 226.*

1. How do muscles and bones work together to move the body?
2. How do bones help the body?
3. What are different ways joints let the body move?

Knee joint

Using Muscles and Bones

1. The muscles in your face help you show your feelings. Think of the different feelings you show using muscles in your face. Move your face muscles to show these different feelings. See how many of your feelings other children can name.

2. You can find out which muscles help you move certain ways. Stand on your toes as shown for as long as possible. Feel which muscles are working. The muscle on the back of your lower leg pulls your heel up. This muscle helps you point your toe. Think of other actions you can do. Guess which muscles you would use when you perform these actions. Then try doing these actions and see if your guesses were correct.

3. Show how you would have to run if you had no knee joints. Then show how you would have to write if you had no elbow joint.

organ (ôr′gən), a group of different tissues that work together to do the same job.

Brain

Nerves

3 How Do Your Brain and Nerves Help You?

The brain is an **organ** inside your skull. It is made up of different kinds of tissues. The tissues all work together so you can think.

Messages go to your brain from all parts of your body. Your brain tells you what the messages mean. If you need to do something, your brain sends messages to your muscles. Your brain tells your muscles how to move.

Messages go to and from your brain over your nerves. Notice the nerves in the picture. Nerves are not all the same size. Some nerves are long and some are short. They go up and down the backbone. Nerves thread their way through most of the body.

What Do Your Senses Tell You?

You have five senses that send messages to your brain. The messages tell about seeing, hearing, touching, tasting, and smelling. For example, nerves in your eyes send messages about what you see to your brain. You do not really see until the messages get to your brain.

The picture shows the senses. What are they? What does each sense tell you?

Think Back • *Study on your own with Study Guide page 226.*

1. What is the job of the brain?
2. How do messages travel to and from the brain?
3. What are the five senses?

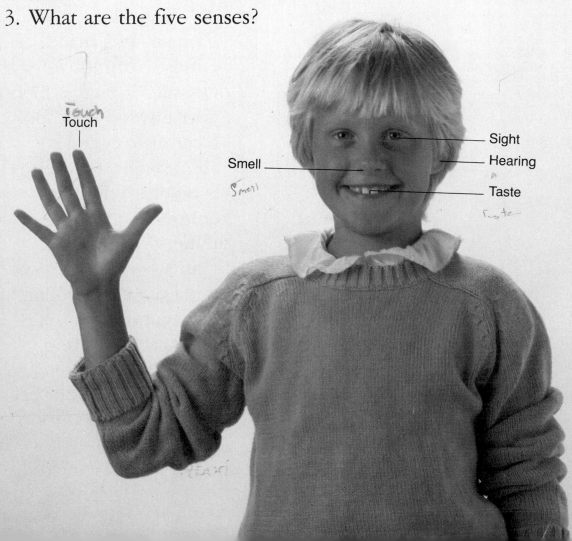

Touch

Smell

Sight

Hearing

Taste

oxygen (ok′sə jən), a colorless gas cells take in to stay alive.

carbon dioxide (kär′bən dī ok′sīd), a colorless waste gas given off by the cells.

Heart

4 How Does Your Heart Help You?

Look at the picture. Notice where the heart is in the chest. Now put your hand over your heart. Can you feel your heart beating?

Your heart beats all the time. It beats about 90 times a minute in a child your age.

Your heart is an organ. It is made mostly of muscle tissue. It pumps blood to all your cells. Blood carries **oxygen** to your cells. Oxygen is a gas that your cells need to stay alive. Blood also carries nutrients from food that your cells need.

Blood picks up a gas called **carbon dioxide** and other wastes from your cells. It carries the carbon dioxide and wastes away from your cells.

Your heart pumps blood into and through little tubes in your body. These tubes are your **blood vessels.** Find the blood vessels in the picture.

Your heart pumps blood to all parts of your body. The blood then travels through blood vessels back to your heart. The blood takes about one minute to travel from the heart and back.

Think Back

• *See Study Guide on page 227.*

1. What is the job of the heart?
2. What does blood carry to the body's cells?
3. What does blood carry away from cells?
4. What does blood travel through in the body?

blood vessel (ves′əl), a tube through which blood travels in the body.

Heart

Blood vessels

5 How Do Your Lungs Help You?

Your heart is in your chest. Your two lungs are also in your chest. The lungs are spongy organs that always have some air in them.

When you breathe in through your nose or mouth, air goes into your lungs. It goes down a long tube to get to your lungs.

Now try this. Put your hands on your chest as shown. Breathe in. What happens to your chest? Next breathe out. What happens to your chest?

Oxygen is in the air that you breathe into your lungs. You know your body cells must have oxygen to stay alive. How does oxygen get from your lungs to your cells?

This boy can feel his chest get larger when he breathes.

78

Your heart pumps blood to your lungs through blood vessels. Find these vessels in the picture. The blood picks up oxygen in your lungs. Then the blood travels back to your heart. Next, your heart pumps out the blood to all of your cells. The blood leaves oxygen in your cells.

The blood picks up carbon dioxide in your cells. It carries the carbon dioxide to your heart. The blood with carbon dioxide then goes to your lungs. Your body gets rid of carbon dioxide when you breathe out.

On Your Own
You know that air goes into your lungs when you breathe. Write a paragraph telling why you think it is important for your lungs to breathe clean air.

Think Back

• *See Study Guide on page 227.*

1. How does oxygen get to the lungs?
2. How do body cells get the oxygen they need?
3. How does the body get rid of carbon dioxide?

Blood vessels

Lungs

Heart

6 How Do Your Stomach and Intestines Help You?

Food tube ——————————

Stomach ——————————

You must eat food to stay alive. Your body must digest the food you eat so that your cells can use it. When your body digests food, it changes the form of the food.

Food starts to be digested in your mouth. Your teeth and tongue chew up the food. Saliva mixes with the food. Saliva is a juice in your mouth. It helps make food soft enough to swallow.

What happens when you swallow the softened food? This food goes down a long food tube to the stomach. Find this tube in the picture. Muscles in the food tube push the food along.

Stomach juices mix with the food. Stomach muscles turn the food around and around. After a while the food looks like a thick liquid. It is now partly digested.

Soon your stomach squeezes out the thick liquid food into your small intestine. The small intestine is a long narrow tube all curled up inside you. Find it in the picture.

Juices in your small intestine finish digesting the food. The thick liquid food is changed to a thin liquid food. Muscles in your small intestine move the thin liquid along. The thin liquid food with its nutrients moves into blood vessels. These blood vessels are in the sides of your small intestine. Your heart pumps the blood with nutrients to all of your cells.

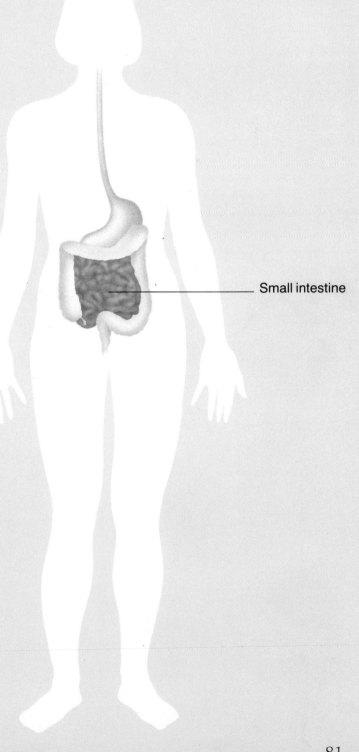

Small intestine

How Does Your Body Get Rid of Food It Cannot Use?

Your body cannot use some parts of the food you eat. For example, your body cannot change fruit skins and seeds to liquid.

Food not used by your body moves from your small intestine to your large intestine. Notice the large intestine in the picture. Your large intestine is a much shorter and wider tube than your small intestine.

In your large intestine, water is removed from food. The parts of the food that are left are wastes. Your body cannot use these wastes. Muscles in your large intestine push the wastes slowly along. After some hours, the wastes are moved out of your body.

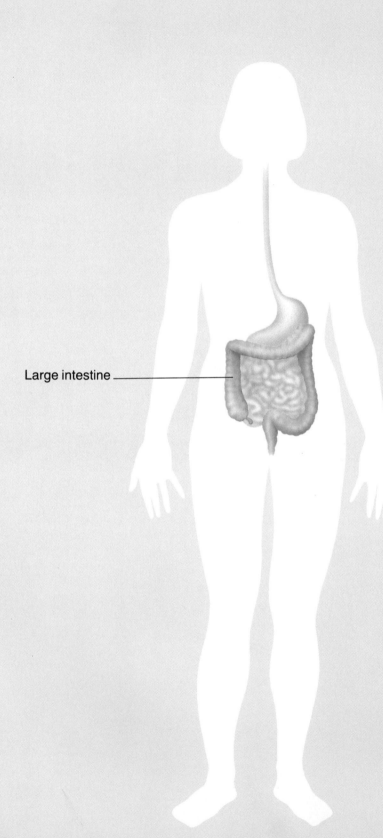

Large intestine

The organs that work together to digest food make up a system. Your body has many systems to do different jobs.

Use a finger to trace the path food takes through the body. Start at the mouth and move your finger down the long tube to the stomach. Then move your finger from the stomach to the small intestine. Follow the twists and turns until you reach the large intestine. Trace along the intestine to the place where wastes leave the body.

Think Back

• See Study Guide on page 227

1. How do the stomach and small intestine help digest food?
2. What is the path that food takes as it is being digested in the body?

What path does food take in the body?

**Finding Out More About Your
Brain, Senses, and Heart**

1. Find out how your brain works when you try to catch something. Throw a ball up in the air and then catch it. Throw a sheet of paper up in the air. Try to catch it. Throw a ball in the air again. Try catching it with one hand, as the picture shows. Do the same thing with a sheet of paper. Which is easier for your brain to think about catching, the ball or the paper? Explain your answer.

2. Find out where the heart is in the body. Put one end of a cardboard tube against a friend's back. Move the tube around until you find the place where you can hear a heartbeat. You will hear a thumping sound: lub-dup, lub-dup, lub-dup. How many times does your friend's heart beat in one minute?

3. See how many things a friend can name correctly using the sense of touch. Ask a friend to close his or her eyes. Touch the friend's hand with a sheet of paper, a cotton ball, a soft brush, and a feather.

Looking at Careers

4. Did you know that pictures can be taken of parts inside your body? A worker called an **X-ray technologist** takes the pictures with an X-ray machine. X-ray machines take pictures of the heart, lungs, and other body organs. They also take pictures of the bones in the body.

An X-ray technologist shows a doctor any X-ray pictures he or she takes. The doctor studies the pictures to see if the body parts are healthy.

Maybe you have had an X-ray picture taken. Explain to the class what happened. You might want to draw "X rays" of parts of the body.

7 How Does Your Body Grow?

Do you know what makes your body grow? You grow because most of your body cells make more cells. Cells grow until they reach a certain size. Then the cells divide to form new cells. For example, bone cells divide to make more bone cells. These new cells also grow and divide. Your body becomes larger as it adds new cells.

You grow in a way that is right for you. No one can tell you exactly how tall someone your age should be. All the children in the picture are the same age, but each is different. Each boy and girl has his or her own way of growing.

You can help yourself grow as you should. Eat healthy foods. Exercise every day to help your muscles get larger and stronger. Get enough sleep each night. Sleep gives your body a chance to rest and grow.

On Your Own
The children in the picture are members of a soccer team. Write a paragraph explaining how playing soccer helps them grow.

Think Back • *Study on your own with Study Guide page 227.*

1. What makes the body grow?
2. What is special about the way a person grows?
3. What can help a person grow as he or she should?

Health Focus

Wilhelm Roentgen's Discovery

About a hundred years ago doctors had no easy way to see inside the body. The only way to see inside was to operate on a patient.

Then in 1895, a German scientist named Wilhelm Roentgen made a wonderful discovery. This scientist discovered X rays. These X rays could pass through the outer layers of the body. The X rays made it possible to see the bones. X-ray pictures gave clear views of the bones.

Today X-ray machines can be used to take pictures of many body parts. X-ray pictures can show the heart, lungs, and other organs. What does this X ray show?

Talk About It

1. What did Wilhelm Roentgen discover?
2. How might Wilhelm Roentgen's discovery help you?

Making Up Riddles About the Body

You have learned something about how your body works. You have also learned something about how your body grows. You can have some fun at home by making up riddles for your family to guess. Make up riddles about parts of the body that you have learned about in this chapter. Look at the examples.

When you breathe in, air comes into them. When you breathe out, air goes out of them. What are they?

Every part of you is made up of them. Your body grows because they divide. What are they?

Reading at Home

Cole, Joanna. *The Magic School Bus Inside the Human Body.* Scholastic, 1989. A classroom experiences first-hand how the body turns food into energy.

Richardson, Joy. *What Happens When You Eat?* Gareth Stevens, 1986. Find out about the processes our bodies go through when we eat.

Chapter 3 Review

Reviewing Lesson Objectives

1. Tell what body cells are. (pages 68–69)
2. Tell what muscles and bones do in the body. (pages 70–72)
3. Tell what the brain and nerves do in the body. (pages 74–75)
4. Tell what the heart and blood vessels do. (pages 76–77)
5. Tell what the lungs do. Tell how cells get oxygen and get rid of carbon dioxide. (pages 78–79)
6. Describe the path food takes through the body. (pages 80–83)
7. Explain what makes the body grow. (pages 86–87)

For further review, use Study Guide pages 226-227

Practice skills for life for Chapter 3 on pages 247-250

SKILLS FOR LIFE

Checking Health Vocabulary

Number your paper from 1–11. Match each meaning in Column I with the correct word or words in Column II.

Column I

1. the smallest living part of the body
2. a group of cells that look alike
3. a place where bones fit together
4. a group of different tissues that work together to do the same job
5. a gas in the air people need to stay alive
6. a gas taken away from the cells by the blood
7. a tube through which blood travels in the body
8. change food to a form that the cells in the body can use
9. a juice in the mouth that helps soften food
10. the organ of the body where nutrients in food enter the blood
11. the organ of the body where wastes are passed out of the body

Column II

a. blood vessel
b. carbon dioxide
c. cell
d. digest
e. joint
f. large intestine
g. organ
h. oxygen
i. saliva
j. small intestine
k. tissue

Reviewing Health Ideas

Number your paper from 1–9. Next to each number write the word that best completes the sentence. Choose the words from the list below.

bones   organ
carbon oxygen
cells   small
heart   tissue
nerves

1. The body is made of many different kinds of _____.
2. Many bone cells together make up bone _____.
3. Two body parts that work together to move the body are muscles and _____.
4. Messages go to and from the brain over _____.
5. The brain is an _____ made up of different kinds of tissues that work together.
6. Blood picks up the waste gas _____ dioxide from the cells.
7. The _____ pumps blood containing oxygen to the cells.
8. Air breathed into the lungs contains _____.
9. Food is changed to a thin liquid in the _____ intestine.

Understanding Health Ideas

Number your paper from 10–18. Next to each number write the word or words that best answer the question.

10. What part of a leg lets it move in different ways?
11. What organ do the five senses send messages to?
12. How does the body get rid of carbon dioxide?
13. How does oxygen get from your lungs to your cells?
14. Where does food start to be digested in the body?
15. How does food get from the mouth to the stomach?
16. What happens to food that the body cannot use?
17. What helps the muscles get larger and stronger?
18. What gives the body a chance to rest and grow?

Thinking Critically

Write the answers on your paper. Use complete sentences.

1. How would your life be different if you did not have one of your senses?
2. In what ways has your body grown since you were a baby?

Caring for Your Teeth

The boy in the picture is telling you the number of primary teeth he has lost. How many primary teeth have you lost? How old were you when you lost each tooth? How old will you be when you lose the rest? This chapter will help answer questions you have about your teeth. You will also learn how to keep your teeth and gums healthy now and in the future.

Health Watch Notebook

Collect pictures of things that help keep your teeth and gums healthy. Combine these pictures together in your notebook.

1 What Are Some Parts of a Tooth?
2 Why Are Primary Teeth Important?
3 What Can Cause Problems with Teeth and Gums?
4 How Can You Keep Your Teeth and Gums Healthy?
5 What Can Help You Choose Good Products for Tooth Care?

1 What Are Some Parts of a Tooth?

What do you know about the parts of a tooth? You can see the **crown** and roots of the tooth in the picture on this page. When you look at a tooth in your mouth, you see only its crown. You cannot see the tooth's roots and other parts.

The crown of a tooth is covered by **enamel** as the picture on page 95 shows. This white covering is the hardest material in the body. A tooth's enamel helps protect it from the wear of chewing.

The roots of a tooth are under the gum. The firm, pink tissue around the tooth is the gum. The roots help hold the tooth in the jawbone. Some teeth have one root. Some teeth have two roots. Other teeth have three roots.

The center of a tooth has blood vessels and nerves. Find the blood vessels and nerves in the tooth. Blood in the vessels carries nutrients and oxygen to the tooth. The blood also carries wastes away from the tooth. The nerves send messages from the tooth to the brain. What kind of messages might the nerves send?

Crown

Root

Enamel

Blood vessels and nerves

Gum

95

How Are Teeth Different?

You have different kinds of teeth. Notice the teeth in the picture. How are they different?

Each kind of tooth does a special job. Teeth at the front and sides of your mouth cut and tear food apart. Teeth in the back crush and grind food into bits.

Think Back • *Study on your own with Study Guide page 228.*

1. What part of a tooth protects the crown?
2. What does the root of a tooth do?
3. What are the jobs of the blood vessels and nerves in a tooth?
4. What are some jobs that different kinds of teeth do?

Different kinds of teeth in the mouth

Teeth that cut food

Teeth that tear food

Teeth that crush food

Teeth that grind food

Learning More About Your Teeth

1. Draw a picture that shows important parts of a tooth, inside and out. Next to each part, write its name.

2. Find the different kinds of teeth in your mouth. Look at your teeth in a mirror as shown. Find the eight teeth with flat edges. Four of these are top teeth and four are bottom teeth. Next find the two top teeth and the two bottom teeth with sharp points. Then look for four top teeth and four bottom teeth with rounded edges.

2 Why Are Primary Teeth Important?

You will grow just two sets of teeth. Right now you have some teeth in your mouth from your first set. You should take good care of the teeth until they are ready to come out.

Your first set of teeth is made up of twenty **primary teeth.** Most babies are born without teeth. You were probably about six months old when you got your first tooth. By the time you were three, you had all of your primary teeth.

Your primary teeth help you in many ways. Primary teeth help shape your face. They help you chew your food. They help you speak clearly. Primary teeth also hold space open so your second set of teeth can come in straight.

Try to take care of your primary teeth. Good care can help keep your primary teeth from coming out too soon. The picture shows about how old you will be when you lose each primary tooth.

Your **permanent teeth** are your second set of teeth. Maybe you first lost a primary tooth at age six or seven. A permanent tooth soon appeared to take its place. In time a permanent tooth will replace each of your primary teeth. Your permanent teeth can last all your life if you take care of them.

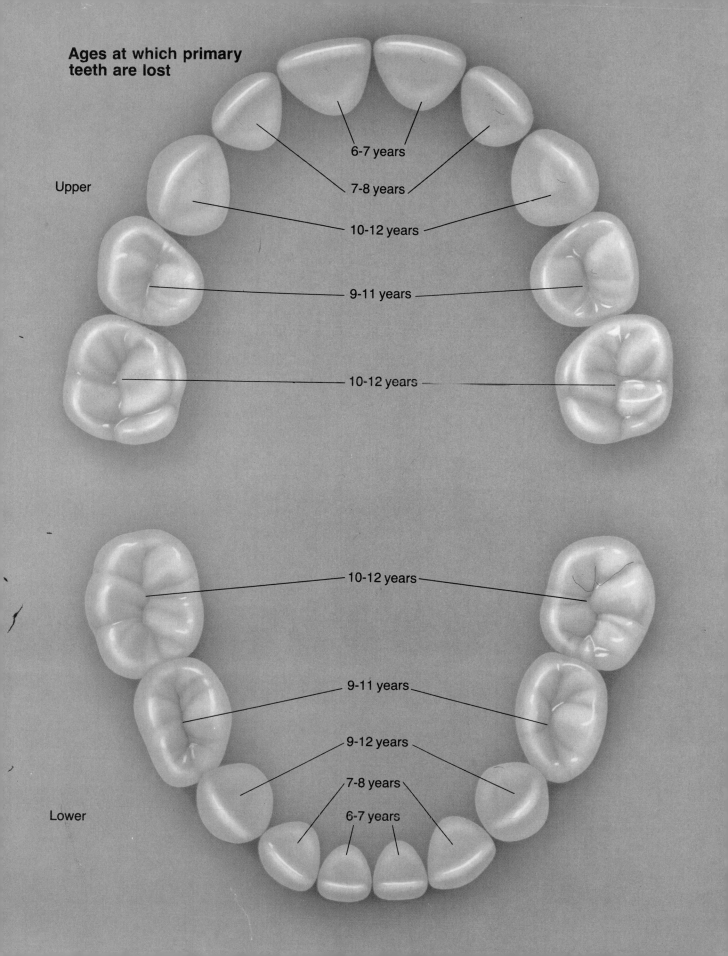

Ages at which primary teeth are lost

Upper

6-7 years

7-8 years

10-12 years

9-11 years

10-12 years

10-12 years

9-11 years

9-12 years

7-8 years

6-7 years

Lower

What Can Help Permanent Teeth Come in Straight?

Suppose a primary tooth comes out too soon. It leaves an empty space. The teeth on each side of the empty space might tip toward the space. The permanent tooth might not have enough room to grow in. It will grow in crooked.

The picture shows an open space after a primary tooth came out too soon. The primary teeth on both sides have tipped toward each other. What will happen to the permanent tooth as it grows in the space?

The permanent tooth does not have enough room to grow in straight.

A dentist can keep primary teeth from moving out of place. The dentist uses the space maintainer you see in the picture. The space maintainer is made of wire. The maintainer holds a space open for the permanent tooth that will grow in later. Then the permanent tooth will have a better chance of growing in straight.

Think Back • *Study on your own with Study Guide page 228.*

1. What are the jobs of primary teeth?
2. What can happen if a primary tooth comes out too soon?
3. How can a dentist help keep primary teeth from moving out of place?

Space maintainer

plaque (plak), a sticky
material made up of
germs.

cavity (kav′ə tē), a hole
in a tooth caused by acid.

3 What Can Cause Problems with Teeth and Gums?

Bumping a tooth on something hard can hurt a tooth. **Plaque** can also hurt a tooth. Plaque is a sticky covering of harmful germs. Plaque is always forming on your teeth and between them. You cannot see plaque but it can still be there.

Many of the foods you eat have sugar in them. The germs in plaque use the sugar to make an acid. In time, this acid can make a hole in a tooth. A hole in a tooth is a **cavity.** You can see a tooth cavity in the picture.

Cavity in a tooth

Plaque can hurt gums as well as teeth. Gum disease begins when plaque builds up where the teeth and gums meet. The picture shows where plaque can build up on teeth. The acid in the plaque harms the gums. If you have gum disease, your gums might bleed when you brush your teeth.

Think Back • Study on your own with Study Guide page 228.

1. How can plaque hurt a tooth?
2. What is a cavity?
3. How does plaque harm gums?

Did You Know?
Once harmful acids form in the mouth, they can attack the teeth for about twenty minutes.

The green dye shows where plaque has built up on these teeth.

4 How Can You Keep Your Teeth and Gums Healthy?

Brushing your teeth helps prevent cavities. You should try to brush your teeth at least once a day. Bedtime is a good time to brush your teeth. Also brush your teeth after eating if you can. Brushing helps remove plaque and bits of food from your teeth and gums.

The pictures show some good ways to brush your teeth. Hold the toothbrush alongside the teeth. Tip the brush back against the gum line as the picture shows. Brush back and forth, back and forth. Brush the outsides and the insides of your teeth. Use short strokes. How will you brush the insides of your front teeth?

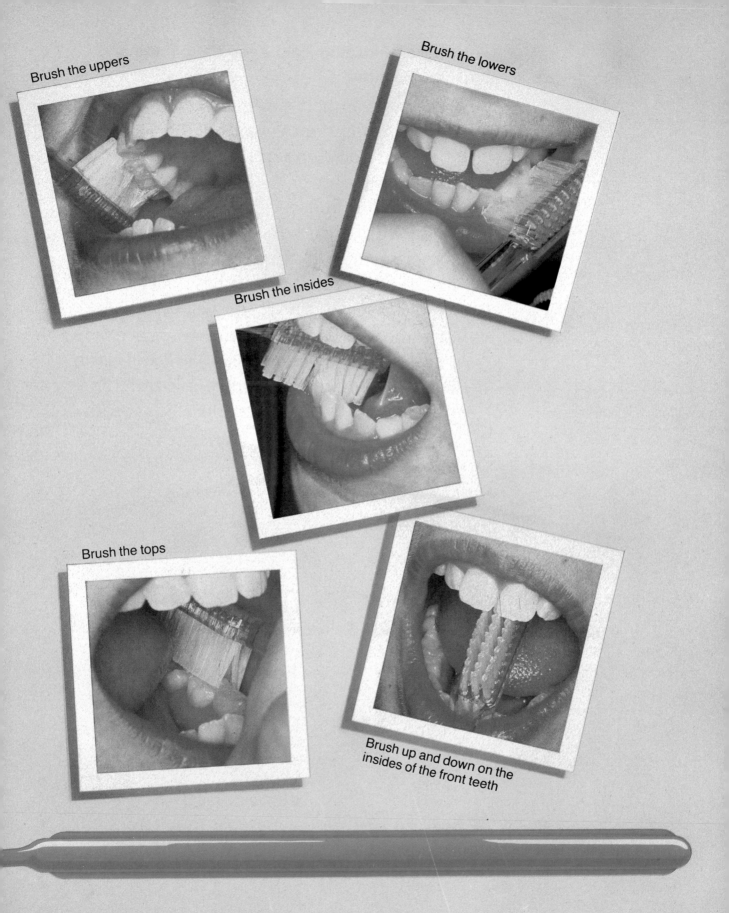

Brush the uppers

Brush the lowers

Brush the insides

Brush the tops

Brush up and down on the insides of the front teeth

How Can Flossing Help Keep Your Teeth and Gums Healthy?

Flossing can help prevent cavities in your teeth. Flossing removes plaque and bits of food from between your teeth and near your gum line. It helps keep plaque from harming your gums.

The boy shown here has asked his mother for help in flossing his teeth. She has carefully placed dental floss between two of his teeth. Next, she will gently move the dental floss up and down the side of each tooth. Gentle flossing will not harm the gums. You might want to ask an adult in your family to help you floss your teeth.

This mother is helping her son floss his teeth.

What Kinds of Foods Can Help Keep Your Teeth and Gums Healthy?

Eat foods from the four food groups each day to help keep your teeth and gums healthy. What foods from the four food groups do you see in the picture?

Try not to eat too many sweet, sticky foods. Caramels, cookies, pies, and cakes are all sweet, sticky foods. Sugar in these foods can stick to your teeth. If you do not brush right away, the sugar can cause cavities.

Suppose you chew gum. What kind of gum can you chew to not harm your teeth?

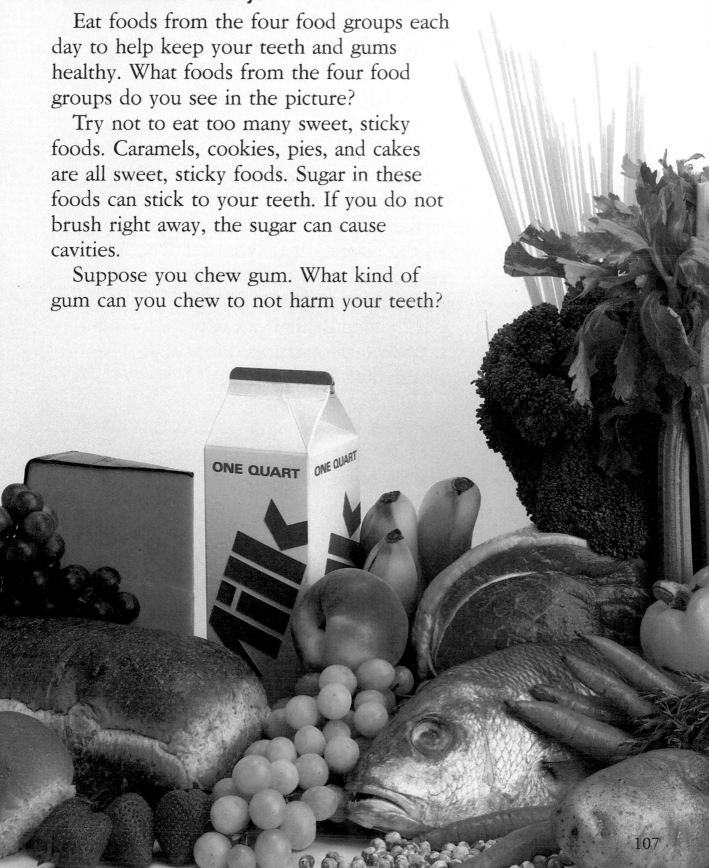

107

How Does a Dentist Help Keep Your Teeth and Gums Healthy?

If you can, visit a dentist as often as he or she tells you. The dentist has special tools to clean your teeth. Sometimes a dental hygienist works in the dentist's office. The dental hygienist can also clean your teeth.

Even if you brush and floss, some plaque might stay on your teeth and harden. The plaque can cause gum disease. You cannot get the plaque off by yourself. The dentist uses special tools to clean the plaque off your teeth.

If the dentist finds a cavity, he or she fills it. Look at the pictures. How does a dentist fill a cavity?

Think Back • *Study on your own with Study Guide page 229.*

1. How can brushing and flossing help keep teeth and gums healthy?
2. What kinds of foods help keep teeth and gums healthy?
3. How does a dentist help keep teeth and gums healthy?

This dentist is getting ready to fill a cavity in the boy's tooth.

The dentist prepares the cavity for filling.

The dentist picks up filling material.

The dentist puts the filling material in the cavity.

The dentist gives the filling material a final polishing.

109

Keeping Teeth and Gums Healthy

1. You cannot do a good job of cleaning your teeth if your toothbrush is worn out. The picture shows how the brush part of your toothbrush should look. Check your toothbrush at home to see if the brush part is worn out. Tell what you might do about your toothbrush if it is worn out.

2. Unscramble these words. Each word has to do with tooth care. Write the unscrambled words on your own paper.

> fsoslnig
> rbuhsnig
> oothtrbuhs
> denalt yhgeinsti

3. Draw pictures of foods that help keep your teeth and gums healthy. Cut the pictures out and paste them on paper to make a design. Put a title on your design such as "Foods to Help Keep Teeth and Gums Healthy."

Looking at Careers

4. A **dental hygienist** works in a dentist's office. She or he uses special tools to clean teeth. A dental hygienist also takes X rays of teeth.

Pretend that you are a dental hygienist working in a dentist's office. Act out what a dental hygienist does. What did you like and not like about being a hygienist?

5 What Can Help You Choose Good Products for Tooth Care?

What can an advertisement do? An ad can tell many things about a product. For example, an ad might tell how to use the product. The ad might also tell what is in the product and how much it costs. What does this toothpaste ad say?

You might see many ads for toothpastes. Most of them say that they help prevent cavities. What can help you decide which toothpaste to choose?

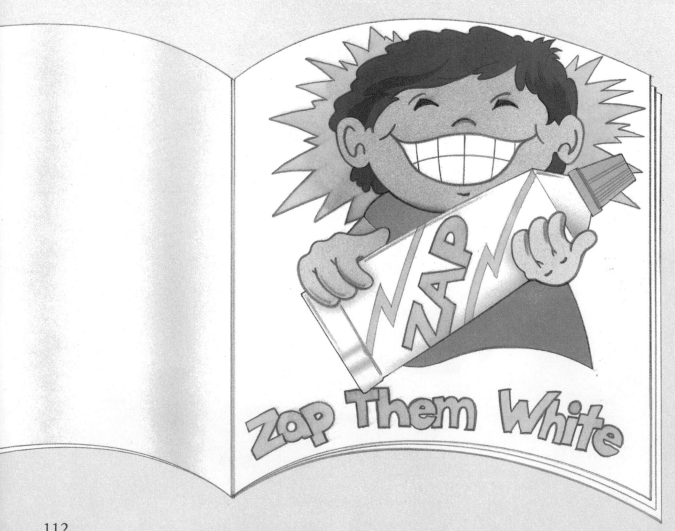

Zap Them White

You can ask dentists or dental hygienists for advice. They will probably tell you to look on a toothpaste box or tube. Look for a special seal. It is the ADA seal you see in the picture. ADA stands for the American Dental Association. The ADA puts its seal on toothpastes that help prevent cavities. Look for the ADA seal when you are choosing a toothpaste.

On Your Own
Make up an advertisement for a toothpaste. Be sure your ad has information about the ADA seal.

Accepted
COUNCIL ON DENTAL THERAPEUTICS
AMERICAN DENTAL ASSOCIATION

How Can You Decide Which Products Are Right for You?

You can ask your dentist or dental hygienist for advice if you need a new toothbrush. Either one can tell you what kind of toothbrush you should use. Then you will be able to choose the toothbrush that is right for you.

Use a toothbrush that is the right size for your mouth. The brush part of the toothbrush should be small enough to reach each of your teeth. The brush should be soft with rounded edges. The top of the toothbrush should be flat, as the pictures show.

This boy's toothbrush is the right size for his mouth.

114

You also can ask your dentist which kind of dental floss you should use. You can choose waxed or unwaxed dental floss, as the picture shows. You might find waxed floss easier to use if your teeth are close together.

Think Back • *Study on your own with Study Guide page 229.*

1. What might an advertisement tell about a product for tooth care?
2. What does the ADA seal on a toothpaste tell about the toothpaste?
3. Who can help people choose good products for tooth care?

Different kinds of dental floss

William Addis's Toothbrush

Suppose you did not have a toothbrush. What would you use to clean your teeth?

Many hundreds of years ago, people did not have toothbrushes. Some people cleaned their teeth by rubbing them with chalk and a rag. Others cleaned their teeth by scraping them with a twig about the size of a pencil. People first soaked the twig in water. Then they pounded the twig on one end until the end looked like a brush.

Many people began using toothbrushes about two hundred years ago because of William Addis. In 1780 he started a company to make toothbrushes. William Addis used ox bones to make the backs and handles of his toothbrushes. The bones were boiled to remove fat and grease. Then the bones were cut in the shape of a toothbrush. Small holes were drilled in the bones. The holes were stuffed with bristles made of white horsetail hair. The picture shows some toothbrushes like the ones William Addis made.

The company that William Addis started is still making toothbrushes. The toothbrushes are no longer made from bone and horsetail hair. Now the handles are made from plastic and the bristles from nylon.

Talk About It
1. How did William Addis make toothbrushes?
2. If you were making a new kind of toothbrush, what would it be like?

Caring for Your Teeth at Home

Talk with your family about ways to help keep the teeth and gums healthy. What can you tell your family about brushing and flossing the teeth?

Maybe you can draw a picture to show your family. Make a drawing that shows something you have learned about caring for the teeth. What does this girl's picture show?

Reading at Home

Dental Care by Brian R. Ward. Watts, 1986. Find out how teeth function and how to care for them.

My Friend the Dentist by Jane Werner Watson. Crown, 1987. Learn with your parents about children's visits to the dentist.

117

Chapter 4 Review

Reviewing Lesson Objectives

1. Tell what the enamel, root, blood vessels, and nerves in a tooth do. (pages 94–96)
2. Tell what jobs the primary teeth do. (pages 98–101)
3. Tell how plaque can harm teeth and gums. (pages 102–103)
4. Tell how brushing and flossing, eating healthy foods, and visiting a dentist help keep teeth and gums healthy. (pages 104–109)
5. Tell who can help advise people about good products for tooth care. (pages 112–115)

For further review, use Study Guide pages 228-229

Practice skills for life for Chapter 4 on pages 251-254

SKILLS FOR LIFE

Checking Health Vocabulary

Number your paper from 1–8. Match each meaning in Column I with the correct word or words in Column II.

Column I

1. the part of the tooth above the gum
2. the hard outer covering that protects a tooth
3. the first twenty teeth that come through the gums
4. the second set of teeth
5. a sticky material made up of germs
6. a hole in a tooth caused by acid
7. strong thread that can help clean between the teeth
8. a person who uses special tools to clean teeth and also takes X rays of teeth

Column II

a. cavity
b. crown
c. dental floss
d. dental hygienist
e. enamel
f. permanent teeth
g. plaque
h. primary teeth

Reviewing Health Ideas

Number your paper from 1–9. Next to each number write the word that best completes the sentence. Choose the words from the list below.

between   plaque
cavities   primary
dentists   size
nerves   teeth
permanent

1. The _____ in the center of a tooth send messages from the tooth to the brain.
2. The _____ teeth hold space open so a second set of teeth can come in straight.
3. If a person takes care of his or her _____ teeth, they can last a lifetime.
4. Plaque is always forming on _____ and between them.
5. Teeth and gums can be harmed by _____.
6. Brushing and flossing teeth can help prevent _____.
7. Dental floss is used to clean _____ teeth.
8. People who can give the best advice about tooth care are _____ or dental hygienists.
9. A person should use a toothbrush that is the right _____ for his or her mouth.

Understanding Health Ideas

Number your paper from 10–18. Next to each number write the word or words that best answer the question.

10. What carries nutrients and oxygen to a tooth?
11. What helps hold the tooth in the jawbone?
12. Where are teeth that grind food found in the mouth?
13. How long should permanent teeth last?
14. What can plaque built up where the teeth and gums meet cause?
15. What can flossing remove from between the teeth?
16. How does eating foods from the four food groups help teeth and gums?
17. What does a dentist use to clean teeth?
18. What do toothpastes with the ADA seal help prevent?

Thinking Critically

Write the answers on your paper. Use complete sentences.

1. What advice would you give about buying a toothbrush?
2. What could help you remember to brush your teeth daily?

5

You and Your Safety

What are these children doing to keep themselves safe? This chapter will help you learn many ways to keep safe throughout your life.

Health Watch Notebook

Ask ten adults, "What was the most important safety lesson you ever learned and why?" Write their answers in your notebook.

---

2 How Can You Keep Safe in a Car?

Suppose you ride in a car that pulls up to the curb. What is the safest way to get out of the car?

You should get in and out of a car on the curb side, as the picture shows. This safety rule helps protect you from other cars in the street.

What safety rules should you follow to help keep you safe in a car? One rule is to lock the doors. Usually a locked door will not open even if someone moves the handle. Locked car doors prevent people from falling out of a car accidentally.

This girl gets out of a car on the curb side to stay safe.

The picture shows the most important rule to follow every time you ride in a car. This rule is to wear your safety belt. You will not be thrown out of your seat if the car stops suddenly.

Another safety rule is to not bother the car driver. How might not bothering the driver help prevent accidents?

Think Back • *Study on your own with Study Guide page 230.*

1. What is the safe way to get in and out of a car?
2. What is the most important safety rule to follow when riding in a car?
3. What are some other safety rules to follow when riding in a car?

On Your Own
You know some safety rules to follow when you are in a car. Which rules can also help keep you safe in a school bus or another bus? Use your own paper, and list other safety rules you can follow in a bus. You might write how the rules can help keep you safe in a bus.

This boy buckles his safety belt when he rides in a car.

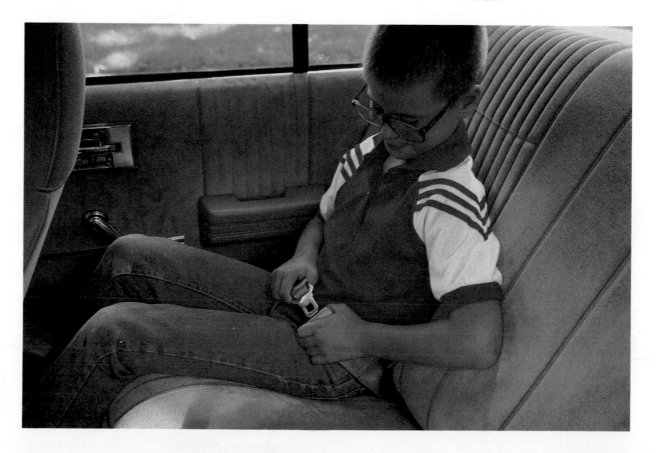

3 How Can You Keep Safe on a Bicycle?

Before you drive your bicycle, check to see if it is safe to drive. Ask an adult to help you. The chart tells you what parts to check.

What can help keep you safe while driving your bicycle? Following these safety rules can help keep you safe.

• Drive a bicycle that is the right size for you.
• Learn how to drive your bicycle well.

Bell

Light

Reflector

Tire

• Learn and use the hand signals for a left turn and a right turn.
• Ride on the sidewalk if your community allows you to.
• Drive on the right-hand side of the sidewalk or street.
• Drive in single file if you are with other bicycle drivers.

Think Back • *Study on your own with Study Guide page 230.*

1. What parts of a bicycle should be checked before driving?
2. What are some safety rules a bicycle driver should follow?

Bicycle Parts to Check

Check the brakes. Be sure they can stop the bike safely.

Check the tires. Be sure they have enough air in them.

Check to see if your bike has a horn or bell, a light, a chain guard, and reflectors.

Reflector

Tire

Chain guard

electric shock, an injury caused by electricity moving through the body.

4 How Can You Keep Safe with Electric Appliances?

Suppose you are making toast. The toast gets stuck in the toaster. How can you safely remove the stuck toast? Unplug the toaster. The picture shows how you should pull the plug. Never pull on the cord. Ask an adult in your family to help you remove the toast. Then you will not burn yourself.

A toaster is an electric appliance. It uses electricity to do a job. Electricity can be helpful, but it can also be harmful. It can cause fires. Electricity can also cause injuries such as burns and **electric shocks.** Handle an electric appliance carefully to stay safe.

Pull on the plug to safely unplug an electric appliance. Never pull on the cord.

Never touch small electric appliances with wet hands. Also, never touch small electric appliances when you are standing or sitting in water. Electricity can travel through the water and give you a shock.

When you finish using a small appliance that heats up, turn it off. Then unplug the appliance. Sparks might come out of the socket if the appliance is not turned off. The sparks can cause a fire. You could get burned.

Think Back • *Study on your own with Study Guide page 230.*

1. What is the safe way to unplug an electric appliance?
2. What are some safe ways to handle electric appliances?

Dry your hands before touching an electric appliance.

129

poison (poi′zn), a substance that if taken into or put on the body can be dangerous to life or health.

5 How Can You Keep Safe with Products Around the House?

People must be very careful when using certain products in their homes. The picture shows some of these products. People use many of these products for cleaning and repairing the home. Which of these products have you seen? The products contain **poisons** that can be harmful.

Many products need to be used only in rooms with lots of fresh air. People can be safe using products that might be harmful by following these safety rules.

• Leave the labels on the products so that people can easily read any warnings.

These products should be used and stored carefully. They contain poisons.

• Read all directions on the label of a product before using it.

• Keep all the products in the containers they come in. Do not put them in different containers.

• Do not mix different cleaning products together.

• Store all the products away from food. Also, store them out of the reach of small children.

• Do not use any of these products alone. Your parent or another adult should be with you.

Think Back • *Study on your own with Study Guide page 231.*

1. Why must people be careful when using certain products around the house?
2. What are some safety rules to follow when using products that contain poisons?

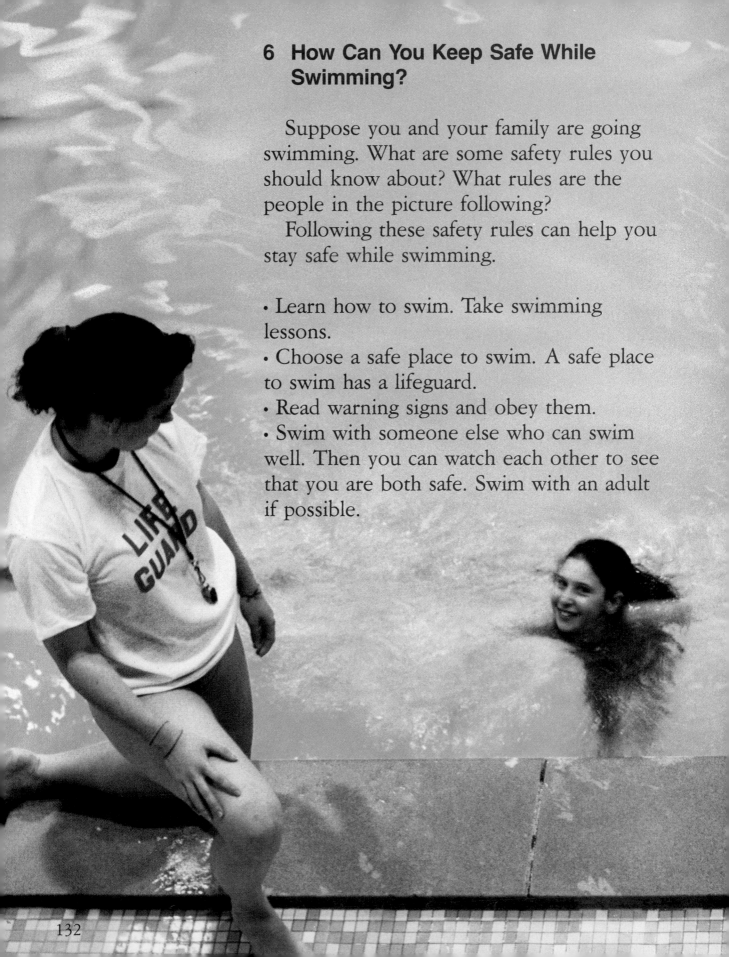

6 How Can You Keep Safe While Swimming?

Suppose you and your family are going swimming. What are some safety rules you should know about? What rules are the people in the picture following?

Following these safety rules can help you stay safe while swimming.

• Learn how to swim. Take swimming lessons.
• Choose a safe place to swim. A safe place to swim has a lifeguard.
• Read warning signs and obey them.
• Swim with someone else who can swim well. Then you can watch each other to see that you are both safe. Swim with an adult if possible.

- Call for help if you need it. Never call for help as a joke.
- Stay out of deep water unless you are a good swimmer.
- Swim only when you feel well. Come out of the water if you feel tired or cold.
- Be careful when you are around water. Do not push or run.

How can following these safety rules help keep you safe?

Think Back • *Study on your own with Study Guide page 231.*

1. What are some safety rules to follow before going swimming?
2. What are some safety rules to follow when swimming?

These swimmers want to swim safely. What ways can they stay safe?

Keeping Safe

1. Solve this puzzle on a sheet of paper. Find out what to do if you are swimming and you see lightning.

C_m_ __t _f th_ w_t_r.
L_ghtn_ng m_ght str_k_ th_
w_t_r.
Th_n _l_ctr_c_ty c__ld
tr_v_l thr___gh th_ w_t_r.
_t c__ld tr_v_l t_ y__ _nd
g_v_ y__ a sh_ck.

2. Explain how following the safety rule shown can help save lives. Draw yourself following another safety rule in a car.

3. Make up a play about the safety rules you should follow while driving a bicycle. Pretend you are talking to young children. What will you tell them?

4. You might like to become a **firefighter** if you think you would enjoy helping keep people safe. A firefighter works to prevent fires. One way a firefighter prevents fires is to make a safety check of a building. Another way is to visit schools and tell about ways to prevent fires. If a fire does happen, a firefighter works to put out the fire. A firefighter also works to save people's lives and homes.

You might want to find a book in the library about firefighters. Find out what a firefighter wears for protection when fighting a fire.

7 How Can You Act Safely to Prevent Injuries from Fires?

What does this family put in their home to help prevent injuries from fires?

Putting one or more smoke alarms in your home can help you if a fire starts. An alarm makes a loud sound when smoke reaches it. An alarm can warn you in time for you to escape a fire without injury. You should leave your home as quickly as possible if a smoke alarm sounds.

Smoke alarms help people stay safe by warning of fires.

Sometimes people are injured when their clothes catch on fire. Stop where you are if your clothes catch on fire. Put your hands over your face to help protect it from flames. Drop down and roll on the floor. Roll to put out the fire and help prevent injuries. The boy in the picture is practicing dropping to the floor and rolling. Practicing helps him remember what to do if his clothes ever catch on fire.

Why should you stop, drop, and roll? You will smother the fire that way. Never run if your clothes catch on fire. Running makes the flames burn more.

Stop, drop, and roll to smother a fire.

137

What Should You Do in Case of a Fire?

Suppose you are in your bedroom when you hear a smoke alarm sound. Leave the bedroom door closed if it feels hot. A hot door means fire is on the other side. Try to get out of the room another way. Leave by a window if possible. Wait on a porch or roof for the fire department.

If you cannot get out of the room, stuff clothes or bedding under the door. This helps keep out smoke and dangerous gases. Then open a window and stay near it. Hold a cloth over your nose and mouth as this girl is doing. The cloth helps keep you from breathing in smoke and gases. Wait for firefighters to come for you.

Suppose the bedroom door feels cool. Then, open the door slowly and crawl out.

Wait near an open window for firefighters if you cannot get out of a room.

Crawling, as shown, helps prevent injuries caused by breathing in smoke and dangerous gases. Smoke and gases rise upward. You will not breathe in much smoke or gases if you crawl along the floor.

Do not go back into your home for any reason once you get out. Call the fire department from a neighbor's home. Look around for family members. They will want to know that you are safe.

Think Back • *Study on your own with Study Guide page 231.*

1. How can a smoke alarm help prevent injuries from fires?
2. What should be done if clothes catch on fire?
3. How can crawling help prevent injuries caused by breathing in smoke and dangerous gases?

This boy is practicing the right way to crawl out of a room during a fire.

8 How Can You Help If an Injury Happens?

You probably try to stay safe when you play. Injuries sometimes happen even when you try to play safely. What should you do if a friend is badly injured while you are playing?

You should follow these rules if someone you are with is injured.

• Stay calm. Try not to get upset. Staying calm helps you think better.
• Try to get adult help. Shout for help. Go for help if no one comes. Tell the injured person where you are going and that you will be back. Try to find a parent or an adult neighbor to help.
• Telephone for help if you cannot find an adult. Some areas have an emergency number that you can call. This number is 911. You can also dial the number 0. An operator will help you if you dial 0. If you have a list of emergency numbers by your telephone, call one of them.
• Speak slowly and clearly when you call to report an injury.
• Listen to any directions that you are given. Follow those directions. Do not hang up the telephone until the person you are talking to hangs up.

The girl shown here is reporting an injury. What is she telling the operator?

This girl is reporting an injury to the operator. She is telling the operator her name, her address, and her telephone number. She is also describing the injury. She will wait to hear what the operator says before she hangs up.

first aid, immediate care given for an injury.

What First Aid Can You Give?

Suppose someone has a small injury such as a small cut. Tell an adult about the injury. How can you help?

You can give **first aid** to others or to yourself for a small injury. First aid is help you give right after an injury.

What first aid can you give for a small cut? First, wash the cut with soap and water. Next, dry the cut with a clean tissue or towel. Then cover the cut with a bandage to help keep the cut clean. Press gently on the bandage if the cut keeps bleeding. The bleeding will soon stop.

Look at the picture. What is the boy doing to help?

The girl's cut has been washed with soap and dried. How will the bandage help the cut?

Sometimes insect bites cause pain, itching, or swelling. Tell an adult about an insect bite that bothers you. The adult can help you if you need first aid.

You should first run cold water over an insect bite to help stop the pain or itching. Then put a cloth with ice on top of the bite. Ice also helps stop pain and swelling. What is the boy in the picture doing for his insect bite?

Think Back • *Study on your own with Study Guide page 231.*

1. How can staying calm help in an emergency?
2. What are some ways to get adult help if someone is injured?
3. What first aid should be given for a small cut?
4. What first aid should be given for an insect bite?

Put ice on a cloth for an insect bite.

Dawnita Reinhardt Works to Help Save Lives

Dawnita Reinhardt always buckles her safety belt when she gets in a car. She knows wearing safety belts helps save lives. She thinks she is alive because she used a safety belt.

Dawnita was in a serious car accident when she was sixteen years old. The police who helped at the accident think that Dawnita could not have lived unless she had her safety belt buckled.

Dawnita Reinhardt now works to help save people's lives. She tells people about the importance of using safety belts. Dawnita gives talks at club meetings about using safety belts. She made a television advertisement about using safety belts. Dawnita also wrote a safety booklet for children. In the booklet, Example Elephant gives children some reasons for using safety belts.

Talk About It

1. How does Dawnita Reinhardt work to help save car riders' lives?
2. What could you do to help save people's lives?

Being Safe at Home

Talk with your family about safety. Talk about ways to help keep the family safe at home.

You might want to make a safety check of your home as this family is doing. For example, you might check if small appliances are unplugged when not being used. What safety check might be made with cleaning products around the house? You might talk over ways to make your home as safe as possible.

Reading at Home

Every Kid's Guide to Responding to Danger by Jay Berry. Childrens Press, 1987. Learn what to safely do in different dangerous situations.

Fire! Fire! by Gail Gibbons. Crowell, 1984. Discover how firefighters battle fires.

Chapter 5 Review

Reviewing Lesson Objectives

1. Tell who is most responsible for a person's safety. (pages 122–123)
2. List some safety rules to follow when riding in a car. (pages 124–125)
3. Tell what should be checked on a bicycle to see if it is safe to drive. List some safety rules to follow while driving a bicycle. (pages 126–127)
4. Tell about some safe ways to handle electric appliances. (pages 128–129)
5. List some safety rules to follow when using products that contain or give off poisons. (pages 130–131)
6. List some safety rules to follow when swimming. (pages 132–133)
7. Tell how injuries from fires can be prevented. (pages 136–139)
8. Tell how to get adult help if someone is injured. Tell how to give first aid for small injuries. (pages 140–143)

For further review, use Study Guide pages 230-231

Practice skills for life for Chapter 5 on pages 255-258

SKILLS FOR LIFE

Checking Health Vocabulary

Number your paper from 1–4. Match each meaning in Column I with the correct word or words in Column II.

Column I

1. damage to the body
2. a substance that if taken into or put on the body can be dangerous to life or health
3. immediate care given for an injury
4. an injury caused by electricity moving through the body

Column II

a. electric shock
b. first aid
c. injury
d. poison

Reviewing Health Ideas

Number your paper from 1–9. Next to each number write the word that best completes the sentence. Choose the words from the list below.

careful   plug
clearly   products
crawl   protect
lifeguard   safety
parts

1. Being _____ can help keep you safe.
2. To stay safe when riding in a car, wear a _____ belt.
3. To keep safe on a bicycle, check the bicycle _____ and follow safety rules.
4. To safely unplug an electric appliance, pull on its _____.
5. Keep all _____ in the containers they came in.
6. To _____ small children, store cleaning products out of their reach.
7. A safe place to swim has a _____.
8. To help prevent injuries caused by breathing in smoke, _____ out of a room.
9. Speak slowly and _____ when telephoning to report an injury.

Understanding Health Ideas

Number your paper from 10–16. Next to each number write the word or words that best answer the question.

10. Who is most responsible for a person's safety?
11. What side of a car is safe to get in and out of?
12. Who should help a child give a bicycle a safety check?
13. What should be read before using any product that contains poisons?
14. How can swimming with someone else who swims well help keep a person safe?
15. What three words should a person remember if his or her clothes catch on fire?
16. How can ice or cold water help an insect bite?

Thinking Critically

Write the answers on your paper. Use complete sentences.

1. What are two safety rules an adult can follow if someone is injured?
2. What is another way fires in home kitchens can be prevented other than using electric appliances carefully?

6

Medicines, Drugs, and Your Health

This person knows a lot about medicines. She knows how different kinds of medicines can help people. She also knows how people can use medicines safely. Some medicines can be harmful if not used correctly.

This chapter will teach you about medicines and how to use them safely. Learning how and when to use medicines can help keep you healthy throughout your life.

Health Watch Notebook

Put ads of different kinds of medicines in your notebook. Underline in each ad where it tells how to use the medicine safely.

1   What Are Different Kinds of Medicines?
2   Why Do People Use Medicines?
3   How Can People Be Safe with Medicines?
4   What Can You Do Besides Using Medicines?
5   What Are Some Harmful Drugs?

What Are Over-the-Counter Medicines?

An **over-the-counter medicine** is another kind of medicine that people use. People do not need a prescription to buy this kind of medicine. Cough syrups and medicines for a fever are examples of over-the-counter medicines. The labels and boxes of many over-the-counter medicines have directions for using the medicines. A pharmacist can also give people information about using these medicines.

Drugstores sell over-the-counter medicines. Some supermarkets and department stores also sell them. What over-the-counter medicines do you see here? What other over-the-counter medicines do you know about?

Think Back • *Study on your own with Study Guide page 232.*

1. How can medicines help people?
2. What is a prescription medicine?
3. What is an over-the-counter medicine?

Stores sell many different kinds of over-the-counter medicines.

UPSET STOMACH PILLS

Aspirin Tablets

Liquid Aspirin

COLD TABLETS

Nasal Spray

vaccine (vak′sēn′), a medicine that can prevent a disease.

virus (vī′rəs), a tiny germ that can cause diseases such as measles, mumps, and polio.

What Are Vaccines?

Vaccines are medicines that can help prevent diseases. Most people get vaccines in shots.

People get vaccines to prevent diseases such as measles, mumps, and polio. Measles vaccine and mumps vaccine are given as shots. Polio vaccine is given as drops in the mouth.

Germs called **viruses** cause measles, mumps, and polio. Viruses are much smaller than bacteria. What kinds of viruses are shown in the picture?

Mumps virus

Measles virus

Polio virus

156

Not all diseases can be prevented with vaccines. Not all diseases can be cured with medicines. But some medicines can help people who are sick start to feel better.

AIDS is a serious disease that is caused by a virus. Some adults get AIDS, but very few children get it. AIDS is not spread by food, water, or air. You cannot get AIDS by touching or being near someone who has it. AIDS cannot be cured with medicines. It cannot be prevented with vaccines. Scientists all over the world are trying to make medicines to help cure or prevent AIDS.

Think Back • *Study on your own with Study Guide page 232.*

1. What ways are medicines used?
2. What kinds of germs cause diseases?
3. How do germs cause a person to become sick?
4. How is AIDS different from many diseases?

AIDS virus

3 How Can People Be Safe with Medicines?

Medicines can harm people if used in the wrong way. People should follow these rules for safety with medicines.

• Only an adult in charge of a child should give the child medicine. The adult should carefully follow the directions on the medicine as this parent is doing.

• Prescription medicines should never be shared. One person's medicine might make another person sick.

• A child should tell an adult in charge about any **side effects** from a medicine. An upset stomach or a headache could be a side effect of a medicine.

• Store medicines in high cabinets, with locks if possible. Then small children cannot reach the medicines or take them.

• Leave the labels on all medicines. People can read the labels to be sure they take the right medicine.

• Keep medicine containers closed. Some medicines have safety caps. Small children cannot open these medicines.

Think Back • _Study on your own with Study Guide page 233._

1. Who can safely give children medicine?
2. Why should prescription medicine never be shared?
3. How should medicines be stored?

This parent is carefully
following the directions
on the medicine.

4 What Can You Do Besides Using Medicines?

When have you seen such advertisements for over-the-counter medicines? The ads usually tell how medicines can help you feel better.

Do you always need medicine to help you feel better? Suppose you have a mild headache. Maybe your head aches a little because you need sleep or food. Sleeping or eating might help you feel better. Often tiny aches and pains soon go away. You do not need medicine for every ache or pain.

This advertisement tells you what this medicine can supposedly do.

Sometimes you might not feel well because your feelings are upset. These feelings might make your stomach hurt. Relaxing might help you feel better. The pictures show some ways to relax. Which of these ways would you use to relax?

People should use medicines only if they really need them. Tell an adult in charge of you if you feel sick. The adult or doctor will decide if you need a medicine to feel better.

On Your Own
Look at the pictures of the ways to relax. Write a story about one of the pictures. Write how a person who has upset feelings might use that way of relaxing to feel better.

Think Back • *Study on your own with Study Guide page 233.*

1. What besides medicine can sometimes help a tiny ache or pain go away?
2. When should a person use medicines?

These ways of relaxing can sometimes help a person who is not very sick feel better.

More About Using Medicines

1. A good way to relax is to breathe in deeply. Hold in the breath and count in your mind to five. Then slowly let out the air. Do this several times.

Find out about some other good ways to relax. You might ask your teacher. You might also ask a parent or an adult in charge of you.

2. The poster shows one way to use medicines safely. Think of other ways to use medicines safely. Make a poster about one of these ways. Hang up your poster to remind people to use medicines safely.

Looking at Careers

3. You might see a **pharmacy assistant** helping a pharmacist in a drugstore. The assistant checks to see if the right person's name is on a prescription medicine. He or she also records the name and number of all prescription medicines.

Many pharmacy assistants learn about their jobs while they work in drugstores. Others learn about their jobs by taking special college classes.

Do you think you might enjoy working as a pharmacy assistant? You might like to talk to a pharmacy assistant at a drugstore. Ask the assistant what he or she likes about the job.

These children are enjoying their healthy drinks.

5 What Are Some Harmful Drugs?

Imagine that you have just finished playing a game with your friends. You feel hot and thirsty. You would like a cool drink. The picture shows some healthy drinks. Which drink would you choose?

Some drinks are not healthy. They contain certain drugs. **Caffeine** is a drug found in several drinks. Caffeine can be harmful. Coffee, tea, cola, and cocoa are drinks with caffeine.

Caffeine speeds up the heartbeat. Too much caffeine makes some people feel nervous or causes some people to lose sleep. Doctors think drinks with caffeine in them are not good for young people.

How Is Alcohol Harmful?

Some drinks contain **alcohol.** This drug is found in drinks such as beer, wine, and liquor. Alcohol can be harmful.

Alcohol in drinks goes to the brain very fast. Alcohol changes the way a person's brain works. A person who drinks too much alcohol can have trouble thinking. The person also can have trouble talking clearly, walking, or driving safely.

Suppose a person drinks too much alcohol. What might happen if he or she tries to drive safely?

Alcohol can harm a person's health. A person who often drinks large amounts of alcohol can damage his or her body.

alcohol (al′kə hôl), a drug that can be harmful and is found in beer, wine, and liquor.

nicotine (nik′ə tēn′), a drug in tobacco that can harm a smoker's heart.

What Is a Harmful Drug in Cigarettes?

Suppose someone asks a person your age to try smoking a cigarette. What should the person do? A wise person will not ever start smoking.

Cigarettes, cigars, and pipe tobacco have a drug in them called **nicotine.** This drug makes it hard for a smoker to stop smoking. The best idea is not to start smoking.

Nicotine can be a harmful drug. It can cause heart disease in smokers. Nicotine makes the blood vessels smaller. The heart must work very hard to pump blood through the smaller vessels. A person can get heart diseases if his or her heart works too hard.

Cigarette smoke can be harmful too. The smoke contains tars and dangerous gases. Tar is a dark, sticky substance. Tar can build up in the lungs of people who smoke for many years and cause lung cancer.

All cigarette packages have a health warning. What does this warning say?

166

Why Do People Decide Not to Use Harmful Drugs?

Many people decide not to use any harmful drugs. They know that such drugs can harm their bodies. They also know how hard it is to stop using certain harmful drugs.

These children do not use harmful drugs. These children enjoy playing together. They do not use drugs to feel part of a group. They want to stay healthy.

Think Back • *Study on your own with Study Guide page 233.*

1. How can caffeine harm the body?
2. How can alcohol harm the body?
3. How can nicotine harm the body?
4. What makes people decide not to use harmful drugs?

These children want to stay healthy so they do not use drugs to feel part of a group.

Dr. Percy Julian and Glaucoma Medicine

Dr. Percy Julian was a scientist. During his lifetime, he discovered how to make many medicines. One of these medicines was for the disease glaucoma (glô kō/mə).

A person with glaucoma has too much pressure inside the eyeball. The extra pressure can injure the eyes.

Eyeglasses cannot help a person with glaucoma. Medicines must be used.

The first glaucoma medicines came from plants. Scientists could not get enough of the medicine from plants for all the people with glaucoma. Then Dr. Julian discovered a way to make medicine for glaucoma. He made enough medicine to help many people. Because of Dr. Julian and the medicines later made by other people, those with glaucoma have the helpful medicines they need.

Talk About It
1. What can help people with glaucoma?
2. How might people's lives be different if Dr. Julian had not discovered a way to make medicine for glaucoma?

Being Safe with Medicines at Home

Talk with your family about safe ways to use medicines at home. You and your family might want to check how medicines are stored in your home. You could also answer the following questions with your family about medicine safety.

• Are medicines stored out of the reach of small children?
• Are medicines stored in the containers they came in?
• Are the labels on medicines?
• Do medicines all have caps on them?

If your family finds problems with medicine safety, discuss what to do.

Reading at Home

The Sick of Being Sick Book by Rob Jovial Stine. Dutton, 1980. Discover ways to feel better without taking medicine.

You Can Say "No" to Drugs! by Gretchen Super. Twenty-first Century Books, 1990. Learn how to be a drug-free kid.

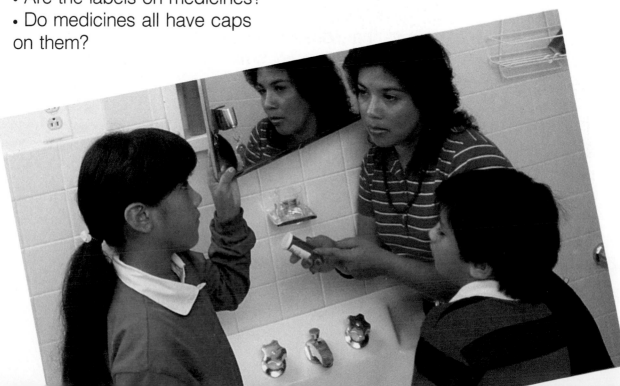

Chapter 6 Review

Reviewing Lesson Objectives

1. Explain the difference between a prescription medicine and an over-the-counter medicine. (pages 150–153)
2. Tell the uses of medicines and tell what causes some diseases. (pages 154–157)
3. Tell how medicines can be used and stored safely. (pages 158–159)
4. Tell what sometimes can be done to feel better without use of medicines. (pages 160–161)
5. Tell how caffeine, alcohol, and nicotine can harm the body. (pages 164–167)

For further review, use Study Guide pages 232-233

Practice skills for life for Chapter 6 on pages 259-262

SKILLS FOR LIFE

Checking Health Vocabulary

Number your paper from 1–9. Match each meaning in Column I with the correct word or words in Column II.

Column I

1. certain living things made of one cell that can cause diseases such as strep throat and tuberculosis
2. a medicine that can prevent a disease
3. a tiny germ that can cause diseases such as measles, mumps, and polio
4. a drug found in drinks such as coffee, tea, cola, and cocoa
5. a medicine that can be bought without a prescription
6. a drug that can be harmful and is found in beer, wine, and liquor
7. a drug in tobacco that can harm a smoker's heart
8. a medicine that can be bought only with a doctor's order
9. an unwanted change caused by taking a medicine

Column II

a. alcohol
b. bacteria
c. caffeine
d. nicotine
e. over-the-counter medicine
f. prescription medicine
g. side effect
h. vaccine
i. virus

170

Reviewing Health Ideas

Number your paper from 1–10. Next to each number write the word that best completes the sentence. Choose the words from the list below.

AIDS	nicotine
drug	pharmacist
bacteria	prescription
labels	vaccines
medicines	viruses

1. Medicines are a kind of _____.
2. A _____ is an order for a medicine.
3. A _____ fills the order for a prescription medicine.
4. Some medicines help cure diseases by killing the _____ that cause the diseases.
5. People get _____ to prevent diseases such as measles, mumps, and polio.
6. Germs called _____ cause measles, mumps, and polio.
7. The virus that causes _____ is hard to get.
8. Leave the _____ on medicines.
9. People should use _____ only if they really need them.
10. Caffeine, alcohol, and _____ are drugs that can harm health.

Understanding Health Ideas

Number your paper from 11–17. Next to each number write the word or words that best answer the question.

11. What kind of medicines can be bought without a prescription?
12. What can some bacteria and viruses cause?
13. Who should a child tell about a side effect from medicine?
14. How can medicines be kept away from small children?
15. What disease has no vaccine to prevent it?
16. What substance in cigarette smoke can cause lung cancer?
17. What do all cigarette packages have written on them?

Thinking Critically

Write the answers on your paper. Use complete sentences.

1. What can people do to stay safe when using medicines?
2. What advice would you give someone who is thinking of smoking a cigarette?

Chapter

7

Your Physical Fitness

This boy is working to become physically fit. You can learn to become physically fit too. In this chapter you will learn several exercises you might do. Being physically fit can help you stay healthy throughout your life.

Health Watch Notebook

Go to the library and find out about two of your favorite sports that are part of the Olympics. Write in your notebook about how these sports help build physical fitness.

1   How Can Being Physically Fit Help You?
2   How Does Having Agility Help You?
3   How Much Exercise Do You Need?
4   How Does Exercise Help Your Body?
5   What Can You Do to Get Physically Fit?

1 How Can Being Physically Fit Help You?

What game are these children playing? What games do you like to play? How can you have fun while you are playing?

If you have **physical fitness,** you can play and work without getting tired easily. Physical fitness can help you have more fun playing games.

Being physically fit can help you look your best. You will have stronger muscles in your back, arms, legs, and over your stomach. Strong muscles help you have good **posture.** Good posture helps you sit, stand, or walk comfortably.

Being physically fit might help prevent heart diseases. Most children do not have a problem with heart diseases. Being physically fit is still important for you. Becoming fit now might help keep you from having heart diseases later in life.

Often, being physically fit can help you do something you have wanted to do. Maybe you wanted to ride a bicycle. You practiced for a long time. How did you feel when you were able to ride your bicycle well?

Think Back • *Study on your own with Study Guide page 234.*

1. What is physical fitness?
2. How can being physically fit help a person?

2 How Does Having Agility Help You?

The picture shows children moving quickly and easily in different activities. They have **agility.** Agility is a part of physical fitness.

When you have agility, you can play games better. What games do you need agility to play? Some people need agility to do their jobs well. For example, people who put up telephone lines need agility.

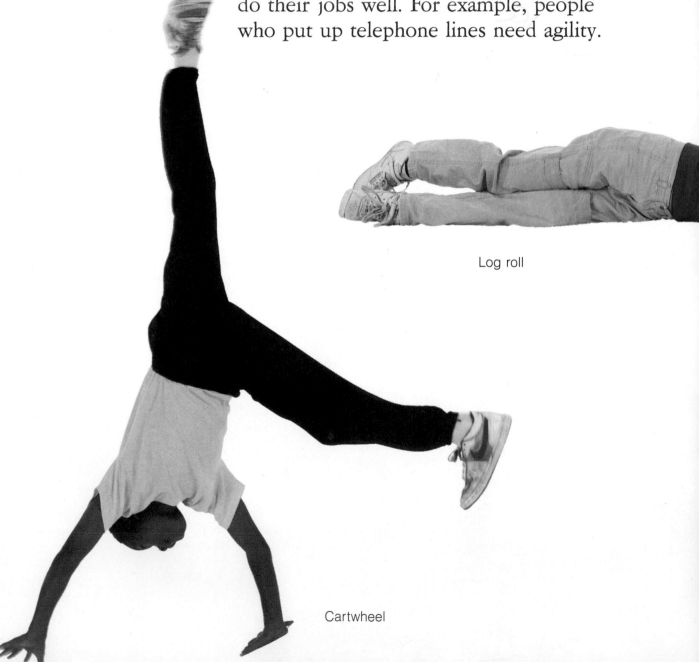

Log roll

Cartwheel

You can do certain stunts to find out if you have agility. You can read about these stunts on page 178. Practicing these stunts can help you improve your agility. Then you can play and work better.

On Your Own
What activity is agility helping each child in the pictures do well? List the activities on your paper and write directions for each activity.

Think Back • *Study on your own with Study Guide page 234.*

1. What is agility?
2. How can having agility help when playing or working?
3. What can improve agility?

Forward roll

Backward roll

177

Finding Out About Agility

1. Try the Half Turn. Stand with your feet apart. Jump in the air as shown and turn while you are jumping. Land facing the opposite direction from which you started. Could you do this stunt easily?

2. Try the Full Turn. Stand with your feet apart. Jump in the air and turn while you are jumping. Land facing the same direction from which you started. Could you do this stunt easily?

3. Try the Heel Click. Jump in the air. Try to click your heels together. Be sure to bend your knees and click the backs of your heels together. Next, jump and try to click your heels two times. Could you click your heels two times?

Half turn

Looking at Careers

4. Do you like to look around in sports equipment stores? Do you like sports that use equipment? Then you might like to be a **sports equipment salesperson.**

One kind of sports equipment salesperson works for a factory that makes sports equipment. The salesperson visits stores that sell sports equipment. The salesperson shows the managers of the stores the sports equipment that the factory makes. The managers can buy the equipment to sell in their stores.

Many sports equipment salespeople learn about their jobs while they are working. Others learn about their jobs when they go to college.

Make a list of the equipment you would need to take part in one sport. You might check to see if the equipment is sold in any sports equipment stores.

3 How Much Exercise Do You Need?

What exercises is the girl doing? How often is she exercising?

Try to exercise several times a day to help yourself stay healthy. When could you exercise during the day? You might exercise in the morning before school starts. Walking to school can be good exercise if you walk fast. You might exercise by playing active games during recess. After school, you might exercise by running or by riding your bike.

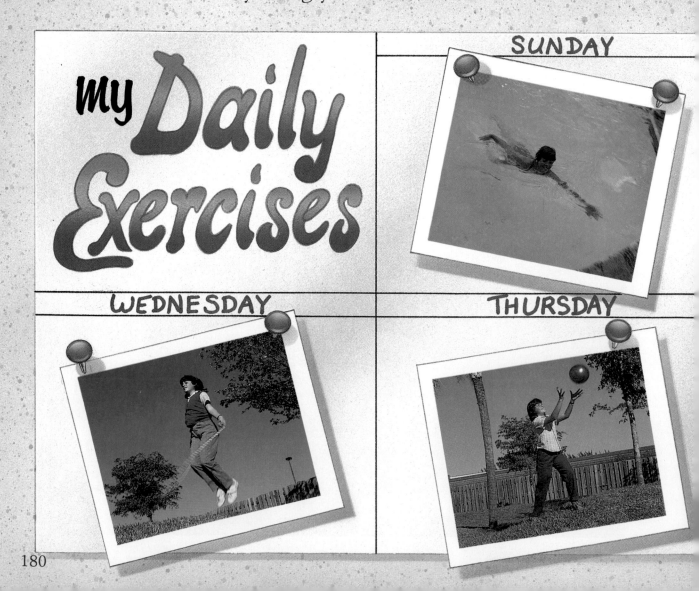

My Daily Exercises

SUNDAY

WEDNESDAY

THURSDAY

Try to stay active for many minutes at a time when you exercise. Exercising for fifteen to thirty minutes at a time helps build physical fitness. Sometimes you might need to rest during exercise. Rest only when you need to. Exercising for at least fifteen minutes at a time is good for you.

Think Back • *Study on your own with Study Guide page 235.*

1. How often should a person exercise?
2. How long should a person exercise at a time?

On Your Own
Lisa wants to improve her physical fitness. Her friend Maria asked her to watch television after school. Her friend Glen asked her to play kickball after school. What do you think Lisa should do? Write what Lisa might say to Maria and to Glen about improving her physical fitness.

MONDAY

TUESDAY

FRIDAY

SATURDAY

4 How Does Exercise Help Your Body?

The muscles in your body become weak if you do not use them. Exercising helps make your muscles strong. Strong muscles give you **strength** for many different activities.

Your body muscles are made up of many muscle cells. Notice the muscle cells in the picture. Your muscle cells get bigger when you exercise. When the cells in a muscle get bigger, the whole muscle gets bigger. Muscles are stronger when they get bigger.

Muscle cell

182

You can do many different activities to make your muscles bigger and stronger. Doing yard work helps build your muscle strength. Doing exercises also helps build muscle strength. What muscles does this exercise help make strong?

Muscles that stretch easily let you bend and move easily. You can do exercises to stretch some of your muscles. Sitting on the floor and touching your toes is a good stretching exercise.

Did You Know?
Not long ago, scientists tested school children of all ages. They found that many children are not very physically fit. The tests showed that these children sit and watch television too much. The children do not get enough exercise. Some of the children decided to change. They decided to become more physically fit by walking more and sitting less.

How Does Exercise Help Your Heart and Lungs?

The girl in the picture enjoys jumping rope. She knows that this exercise will help parts of her body work better. What are these parts?

The heart is one part of the body that exercise can help work better. Your heart is a muscle. Making your heart stronger can help you stay healthy and help keep you from having heart diseases later in life. Exercise helps your heart get stronger. Your heart beats faster during exercise. When you exercise, you help make your heart stronger.

Something else happens when you exercise to strengthen your heart. Your lungs also work better. You breathe more air into your lungs as you exercise. Breathing in more air helps your lungs work better.

You make your heart and lungs work better when you exercise. What activities could you do to help your heart and lungs work better? You could ride a bicycle. You could run or go swimming.

Think Back • *Study on your own with Study Guide page 235.*

1. How does exercise make the muscles strong?
2. What can muscles that stretch easily help a person do?
3. How does exercise help the heart and lungs?

5 What Can You Do to Get Physically Fit?

Following a daily exercise plan can help you become physically fit. A good exercise plan should have exercises to make your muscles strong. It should also have exercises to make your heart and lungs work better. You might want to use the exercise plan shown on pages 188 to 193.

You should warm up your muscles before exercising, as these children are doing. You should also cool down your muscles after you exercise. Warming up and cooling down your muscles helps keep them from hurting. Stretching your muscles is a good way to warm up or cool down.

Warm up before exercising.

Follow these rules to help keep safe when you exercise.

• Choose a safe place to exercise. Be sure you have enough room to move about.
• Ask a responsible adult to show you the right way to do an exercise. Some exercises can be harmful if not done correctly.
• Wear exercise clothes that let you move freely. Keep your shoes tied. You could trip over an untied shoelace.

On Your Own
What rules are the children in the picture following to stay safe when exercising? Write the rules on your paper.

Think Back • *Study on your own with Study Guide page 235.*

1. What kinds of exercises should a good exercise plan have?
2. What can help keep muscles from being hurt during exercise?
3. What are some safety rules to follow when exercising?

project keep fit

Project Keep-Fit is an exercise program that is fun to do. Following this program every day can help you stay physically fit. Be sure to have your teacher help you learn how to do these exercises correctly. Check with your parent or guardian to find out if there is any medical reason why you should not do some of these exercises.

Warm-Up

Side Stretcher
With feet apart, reach down with one hand. Reach over your head with the other hand. Reach a little farther and hold for six to ten seconds. Repeat on other side. Do as many as you can up to three.

Leg Stretcher
Stand facing a wall about an arm's length away. Lean forward bending your arms until your elbows touch the wall. Keep your feet on the floor. Hold for six to ten seconds. Then straighten up. Do as many as you can up to three.

Workout

1. Butterfly with Hop

Stand with your feet together and your arms out to your sides. Hop once and swing your arms up and over your head. Hop again and lower your arms back out to your sides. Stay in one place while you hop. Do as many as you can up to fifteen without stopping.

2. Butterfly with Straddle Hop

Stand with your feet together and your arms out to your sides. Swing your arms up and over your head and hop landing with your feet apart. Hop again, bringing your feet back together and your arms out to your sides. Do as many as you can up to fifteen without stopping.

3. Butterfly with One-Foot Hop

Stand on one foot with your arms out to your sides. Hop on one foot and swing your arms up and over your head. Hop again and lower your arms back out to your sides. Try to repeat the movement on the other foot. Do as many as you can up to fifteen.

4. Jackknife with Hop

Stand with your feet together and arms stretched forward at shoulder height. Jump up and swing your arms up and over your head. Jump again and lower your arms back to shoulder height. Do as many as you can up to fifteen without stopping.

5. Jackknife with Straddle Hop

Stand with your feet together and arms stretched forward at shoulder height. Jump up, swinging your arms up and over your head. Land with your feet apart. Jump again, bringing your feet back together and your arms back to shoulder height. Do as many as you can up to fifteen without stopping.

6. Jackknife with One-Foot Hop

Stand on one foot with your arms stretched forward at shoulder height. Hop on one foot and swing your arms up and over your head. Hop again and lower your arms back to shoulder height. Try to repeat the movement on the other foot. Do as many as you can up to fifteen without stopping.

Cool-Down

Do the stretching exercises on page 188 to help prevent sore muscles.

191

**Keeping Fit While
You Play**

Keep Fit While You Sit

The Twist
Sit and hold your arms out at shoulder height. Turn to the left as far as you can. Stretch your arm muscles. Next turn to the right as far as you can. Stretch your arm muscles. Hold each stretch while you count to ten. Do as many as you can up to three.

The Push and Pull
Sit with your hands together in front of you. Push your hands together as hard as you can while you count to ten. Next grip your hands and fingers and try to pull them apart while you count to ten. Do as many as you can up to three.

Tiffany Chin and Physical Fitness

Tiffany Chin is a champion ice skater. You can see in the picture the strong muscles in her legs. These strong muscles give her the strength to leap when she skates.

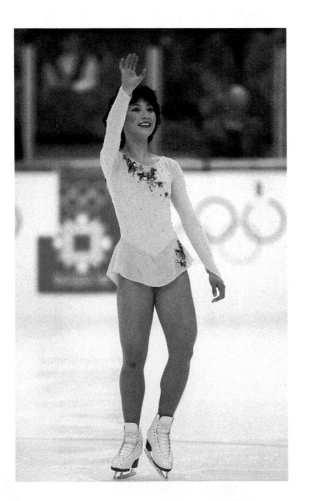

This young skater also needs agility to skate well. She moves quickly and easily on the ice. Because she has agility, she can dance to lively music while she skates.

Tiffany Chin practices skating about four hours every day. Practicing helped her become a great ice skater. Practicing also keeps her physically fit.

Tiffany Chin is one of the best ice skaters in the United States. She has skated in the Olympic games. She has won many medals. She hopes someday to be the best ice skater in the world.

Talk About It
1. How does practicing ice-skating help Tiffany Chin?
2. What sport could you practice to help keep yourself physically fit?

Family Fitness

You might ask some family members to exercise with you at home as this family is doing. Any family member over thirty-five might need to have a health checkup before beginning an exercise program. Maybe you could use the exercises on pages 188–193.

Different family members could take turns leading the group. The leader could tell the others what movements to do. For example, the leader might say this: "Hop five times on your left foot. One, two, three, four, five. Hop five times on your right foot. One, two, three, four, five. Now repeat."

Reading at Home

Three Cheers for Errol! by Babette Cole. Putnam, 1988. Read about Errol the rat who uses his brain and his athletic ability when he competes in the Ratathalon.

Fun with Fitness by Alison Jane Roberts. Hayes, 1987. Shows how to plan a workout routine including exercises for strength and endurance.

Chapter 7 Review

Reviewing Lesson Objectives
1. Tell how being physically fit can help a person. (pages 174–175)
2. Tell how having agility helps in play or work. (pages 176–177)
3. Tell how often and how long a person should exercise. (pages 180–181)
4. Tell how exercise helps the body work better. (pages 182–185)
5. Tell what kinds of exercises a good exercise plan should have. (pages 186–187)

For further review, use Study Guide pages 234-235

Practice skills for life for Chapter 7 on pages 263-268

SKILLS FOR LIFE

Checking Health Vocabulary
Number your paper from 1–4. Match the meaning in Column I with the correct word or words in Column II.

Column I
1. being strong and able to do many different physical activities
2. the way a person holds his or her body
3. the ability to move quickly and easily
4. the ability to exercise without getting tired or injured easily

Column II
a. agility
b. physical fitness
c. posture
d. strength

Number your paper from 5–8. Next to each number write the word or words from the list below that best complete each sentence.

cool down   heart
exercise   warm up

A good (5)＿＿ plan has exercises to make muscles strong and the (6)＿＿ and lungs work better. It begins with a (7)＿＿ and ends with a (8)＿＿ .

196

Reviewing Health Ideas

Number your paper from 1–8. Next to each number write the word that best completes the sentence. Choose the words from the list below.

agility   fit   heart
cells   fitness   safe
exercise   harmful

1. Physical _____ can help a person play and work without getting tired easily.
2. People who have _____ move quickly and easily.
3. Try to _____ for at least fifteen minutes at a time.
4. Running, swimming, and riding a bicycle are activities that can help the _____ work better.
5. Muscle _____ get bigger when a person exercises.
6. Following a daily exercise plan can help a person become physically _____.
7. Learn the right way to do an exercise. Some exercises can be _____ if not done correctly.
8. Choose a _____ place to exercise.

Understanding Health Ideas

Number your paper from 9–15. Next to each number write the word or words that best answer the question.

9. What helps a person have good posture?
10. What can a person do better if he or she has agility?
11. What might be a good exercise to do after school?
12. How does exercising help the lungs?
13. What can help stretch muscles so that a person can bend and move easily?
14. What should a person do before exercising to keep from hurting muscles?
15. What should a person do after exercising to keep from hurting muscles?

Thinking Critically

Write the answers on your paper. Use complete sentences.

1. What different ways do you build your own physical fitness each day?
2. How could improving your agility help you?

Chapter

8

A Healthy Community

These children are helping keep their community healthy. This chapter can help you learn how to keep your community healthy too. You will also learn how community workers help keep a community healthy.

Health Watch Notebook

Collect or draw pictures in your notebook of things that can pollute a community. Under each picture, write a sentence that tells how a community can work to reduce this pollution.

1   What Does a Healthy Community Have?
2   Who Helps Keep a Community's Food Safe to Eat?
3   Who Helps Keep a Community's Air Safe to Breathe?
4   Who Helps Keep a Community's Water Safe to Drink?
5   How Do Sanitation Workers Help a Community?
6   How Can You Help Your Community?

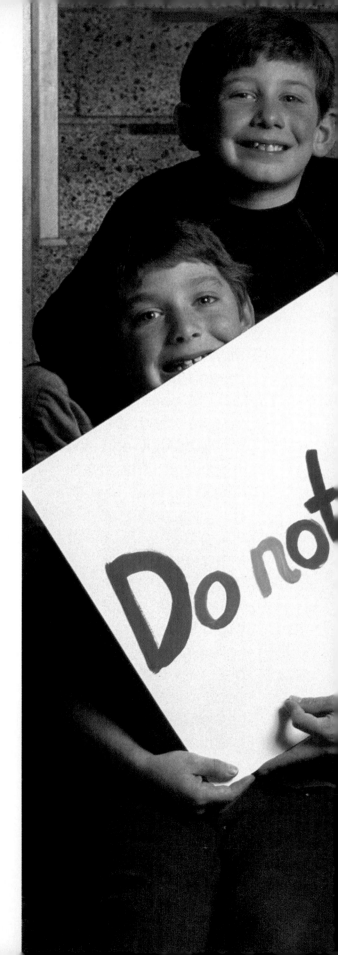

On Your Own
List the places the picture shows that help people in a community stay healthy. Then add three more.

A community has many things people need to stay healthy. A community has places for people to live. It has places for people to work. It has places for people to shop for food and other things. Usually, a community has parks and other places to have fun. Which of these things do you see in this community?

People often need the help of others to stay healthy. Most communities have health workers who can give people this help. For example, doctors and dentists help people stay healthy. Nurses and hospital workers also help people stay healthy. Who are some other health workers?

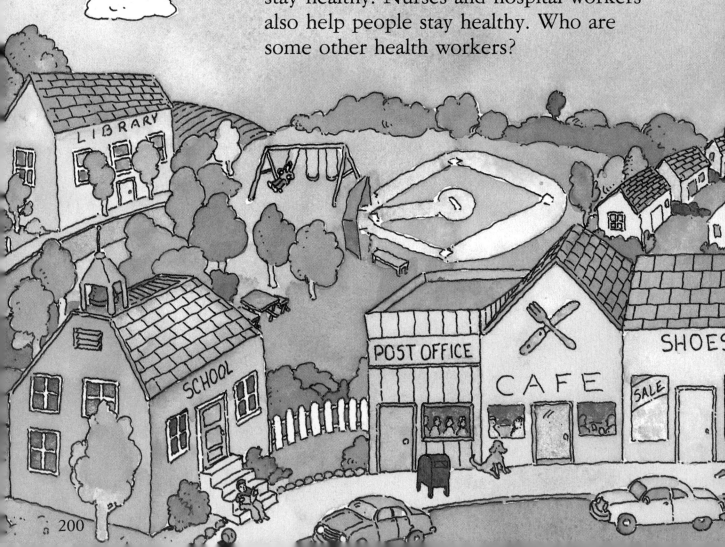

Many communities have a health department. Workers in a health department help protect people from disease. Some workers help make sure that people have clean, safe food to eat. Some workers see that water is safe to drink. Other workers try to solve the problem of dirty air.

Some communities have health department **clinics.** People can get health care sometimes free or at a low cost at these places.

clinic (klin´ik), a place where people can get health care.

Think Back • *Study on your own with Study Guide page 236.*

1. What does a community have that people need to stay healthy?
2. How do health department workers help a community?

2 Who Helps Keep a Community's Food Safe to Eat?

People in a community need clean, safe food to eat. How is a community's food kept clean and safe?

Health workers called **sanitarians** check the food in a community. Sanitarians check to see if food is clean and safe to eat. They check the food in restaurants, food stores, dairies, and food factories.

Sanitarians report any problems they find to the community health department. The department might close a place that does not have clean and safe food to eat.

Sanitarians check food for harmful germs. Some germs that cause disease can grow in food. People might get sick if they eat food with harmful germs.

Sanitarians also check to see if food is prepared in safe ways. Some foods need to be cooked at certain temperatures to kill germs in the food. Sanitarians check to see if these foods are cooked at the right temperatures.

Sanitarians make sure that kitchens are clean. They check to see if food workers have a place to wash their hands. Washing hands with soap and water helps remove dirt and germs from hands. Workers with unclean hands might spread harmful germs to food they handle.

How are these sanitarians making sure that food is clean and safe to eat?

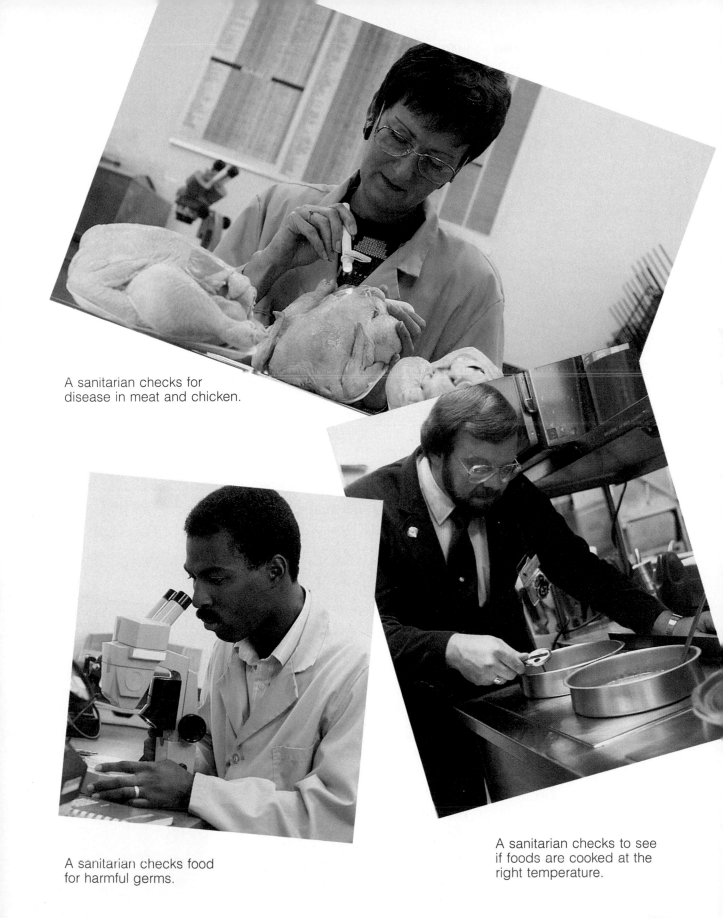

A sanitarian checks for
disease in meat and chicken.

A sanitarian checks food
for harmful germs.

A sanitarian checks to see
if foods are cooked at the
right temperature.

203

What Are Safe Ways to Store Food?

Sanitarians check to see if food is stored in safe ways. Storing foods safely helps keep germs from growing in them. Then people will not get sick from eating foods with harmful germs.

Storing some foods at cold temperatures helps keep them safe to eat. Germs will not grow quickly in foods that are kept cold.

Storing foods in clean containers helps keep them safe to eat. Clean containers have few harmful germs that could get into the foods.

How are these sanitarians making sure that foods are stored safely?

Think Back • *Study on your own with Study Guide page 236.*

1. How do sanitarians help keep food in a community safe to eat?
2. Why must food be prepared in safe ways?
3. Why must food be stored in safe ways?

A sanitarian checks milk containers to make sure that they are clean. What might happen to the milk if the containers are not clean?

204

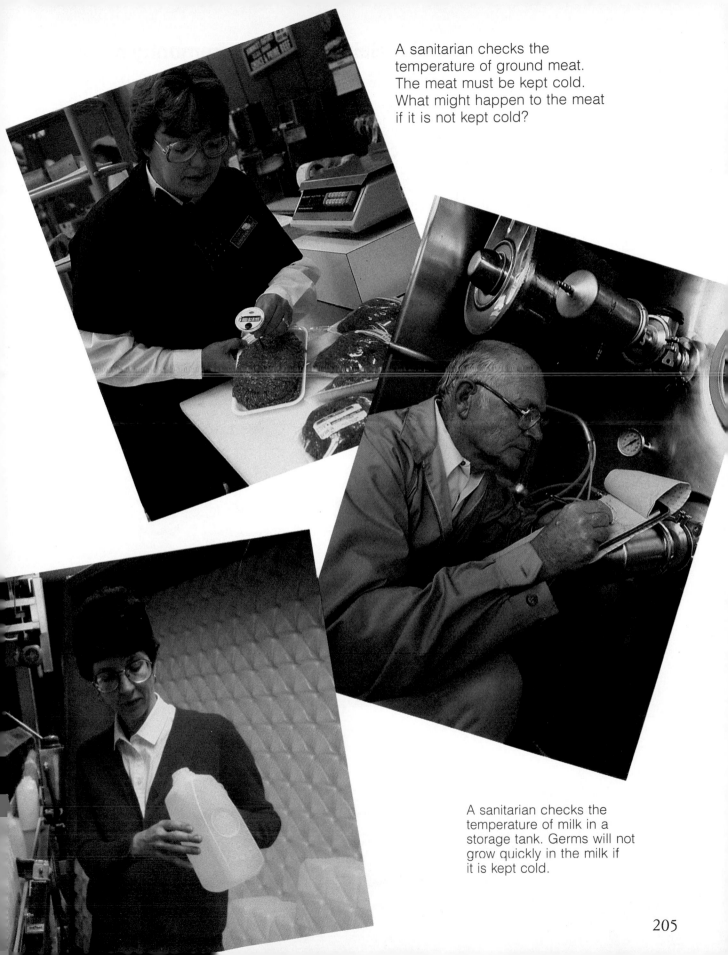

A sanitarian checks the temperature of ground meat. The meat must be kept cold. What might happen to the meat if it is not kept cold?

A sanitarian checks the temperature of milk in a storage tank. Germs will not grow quickly in the milk if it is kept cold.

air pollution
(pə lü′shən), materials in the air that are harmful to health when breathed in.

3 Who Helps Keep a Community's Air Safe to Breathe?

Some health department workers help keep a community's air clean and safe to breathe. They check for **air pollution** in the community. Air pollution is dirt and other harmful materials in the air. People can get sick from air pollution.

The workers report any air pollution they find to the health department. The health department helps the community make plans to stop the pollution.

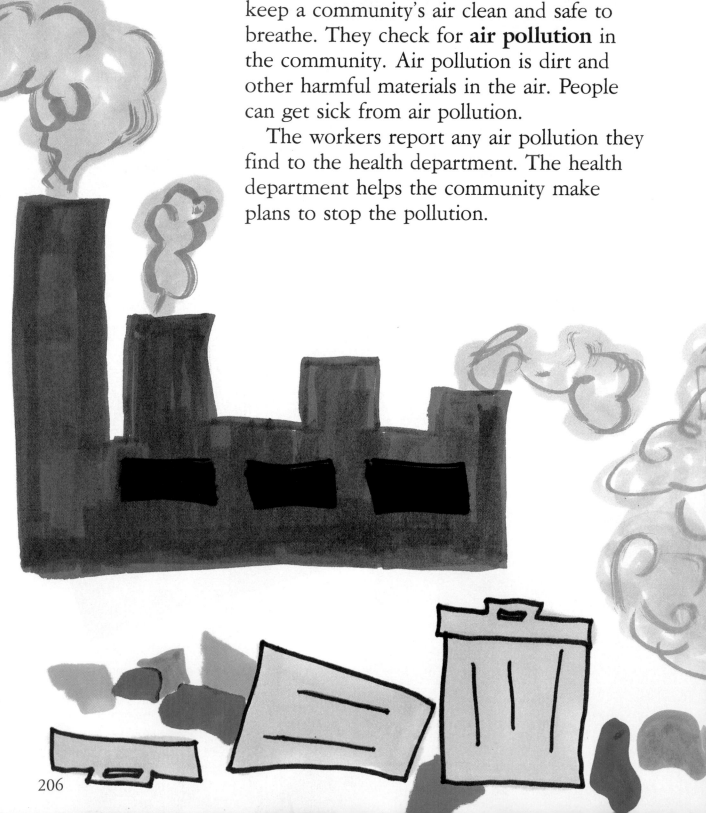

Most air pollution comes from burning. Smoke and other harmful gases go into the air. The smoke and harmful gases make the air dirty. They **pollute** the air. Gases from fuel burned in cars and trucks cause much air pollution.

Some children made the picture you see here. What does the picture show about air pollution?

pollute (pə lüt′), to make dirty.

Think Back • *Study on your own with Study Guide page 236.*

1. Why do people need clean air to breathe?
2. How do health department workers help keep the air clean?
3. What causes air pollution?

4 Who Helps Keep a Community's Water Safe to Drink?

Drinking polluted water can make people sick. What can a community do to make sure its water is safe to drink?

Most communities have a water-treatment plant. Water from a river or lake first goes through pipes to the plant. Workers in the plant make the water safe to drink. Then the water is sent through smaller pipes into buildings.

Health department workers test water from the water-treatment plant. They test to see if the water is safe to drink. They report any water pollution they find to the health department. **Water pollution** is harmful materials in water. The health department makes sure the harmful materials are taken out of the water.

Health department workers also test water that people swim in. They check to see if it is safe for swimming. People can get sick from swimming in polluted water.

This health department worker tests water in a public pool. He also sends some water to a laboratory for more tests. The tests show if the water is safe for swimming.

The workers report to the health department any water pollution that they find. The department might put up a sign where water is polluted. The sign might say NO SWIMMING HERE.

What is the health department worker doing to help keep water safe for swimming?

Think Back • *Study on your own with Study Guide page 237.*

1. What do many communities have to make their water safe to drink?
2. How do health department workers help keep water safe to drink?
3. How do health department workers help keep water safe to swim in?

5 How Do Sanitation Workers Help a Community?

A clean community is a healthy place to live. Garbage is picked up often in a clean community. Garbage will look and smell terrible if it is not collected often. Rats and flies can live in garbage left lying around. The rats and flies can spread harmful germs.

Sanitation workers help keep a community clean and safe. They collect garbage in special trucks. Look at the pictures. What happens to the garbage in different communities?

Think Back • *Study on your own with Study Guide page 237.*

1. Why should a community's garbage be collected often?
2. How do sanitation workers help keep a community clean and safe?
3. Where might sanitation workers take a community's garbage?

Sanitation workers collect garbage that nobody wants. They load the garbage into the back of a garbage truck.

Special equipment inside the truck mashes the garbage and pushes it back into the truck.

In some communities, garbage trucks take garbage to places called landfills. The garbage is dumped there. Then bulldozers flatten it. Finally, bulldozers bury the garbage.

In some communities, garbage is taken to be burned in large furnaces called incinerators.

Learning More About a Community

1. Make a model of a community like the one shown. You might want to use cardboard boxes, clay, and toy objects to make your community. Show what a community has to help people stay healthy. Place your community where others can see it.

2. Find the mystery message. It tells something about pollution. Read the lines from left to right. The letters make a sentence. What is the sentence?

C A R S M A
K E M U C H
A I R P O L
L U T I O N

3. Find out where the sanitation workers in your community take the garbage they collect. You might ask your teacher or parent to help you. You could look under Garbage Collection in the yellow pages of a community telephone book. Then draw pictures to show what happens to the garbage.

 Looking at Careers

4. **Public health nurses** work for a community's health department. They help care for people in a community in many different ways.

Some public health nurses visit schools and help care for children. Some go into homes and help families with health problems. A public health nurse might show a family how to care for someone who is sick. He or she might show a family how to take care of a newborn baby. What is this public health nurse doing? Write a story explaining what the nurse is doing.

Would you like to become a public health nurse? If so, you need to go to college between two and four years.

6 How Can You Help Your Community?

On Your Own
Write a story telling how the family in the picture is helping their community.

litter, trash that is not thrown away as it should be.

recycle (rē sī′kəl), to use something over again.

The people in the picture are helping their community. How are they helping?

You can help your community by not leaving any **litter** lying around. Litter is trash that is not thrown away as it should be. Litter can make a community dirty and unattractive. Litter can cause health problems. For example, a person could get cut by broken glass left in the grass. Throw away all litter correctly. Put it in a covered can or in a plastic bag that closes tightly.

You can help your community by using some things over again. For example, you can use clean paper bags more than once. Your community will have less trash to get rid of if you use things again. You **recycle** things when you use them again.

Your community might have a recycling center. You can collect cans, glass bottles, and newspapers and bring them to a center. These objects can be recycled to make new cans, bottles, and paper.

Think Back • *Study on your own with Study Guide page 237.*

1. How can not leaving litter lying around help a community?
2. How can recycling things help a community?

Helping the Green Bay Community

The school children in Green Bay, Wisconsin, plant trees each year to help their community. The trees help the community look beautiful. They also help the community have less air pollution.

Planting groups of trees can help make city air less polluted. The leaves on trees help take pollution out of the air. Tiny hairs on the outsides of the leaves trap bits of pollution in the air. The bits of pollution stay on the leaves until rain washes them off.

The children in Green Bay first started planting trees in 1964. The children buy young trees from the city at a low cost. They plant the trees in late spring. Since 1964, the children have planted over 60,000 trees.

Talk About It

1. How do the trees that children in Green Bay plant help keep the air clean?
2. How could you help keep the air in your community clean?

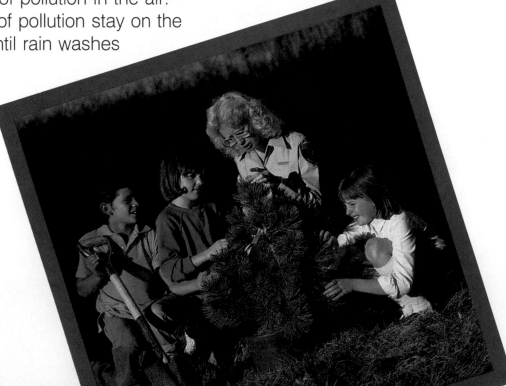

Helping Your Community

What can you tell your family about sanitation workers? How can you and your family help these workers?

You can help the sanitation workers in your community have less trash to pick up. Recycle old clothes, books, and toys. Do not throw them out.

You could save newspapers and bring them to recycling centers. The papers can be taken to factories. Old papers get made into new papers at these factories.

You could also save glass bottles, metal cans, and plastic containers. Then bring the items to a recycling center. The items can be recycled to make new bottles, cans, and containers.

Reading at Home

A Day in the Life of a Medical Detective by Adam Carter. Troll, 1985. Follow an epidemiologist through a day at work.

Kids and Communities by Kathy Darling. Monday Morning, 1989. Learn how you can contribute to the needs of your community.

Chapter 8 Review

Reviewing Lesson Objections

1. Tell what a community has to help keep people in the community healthy. (pages 200–201)
2. Tell how sanitarians work to help keep food in a community clean and safe to eat. (pages 202–205)
3. Tell how some health department workers help keep a community's air safe to breathe. (pages 206–207)
4. Tell how some health department workers help keep a community's water safe to drink. (pages 208–209)
5. Tell how sanitation workers help keep a community clean and safe. (pages 210–211)
6. Tell what people can do to help keep themselves and their community healthy. (pages 214–215)

For further review, use Study Guide pages 236-237

Practice skills for life for Chapter 8 on pages 267-269

SKILLS FOR LIFE

Checking Health Vocabulary

Number your paper from 1–8. Match each meaning in Column I with the correct word or words in Column II.

Column I

1. a place where people live, work, shop, and play
2. a place where people can get health care
3. a person who checks to see if food is clean and safe to eat
4. materials in the air that are harmful to health when breathed in
5. to make dirty
6. materials in water that are harmful to health
7. trash that is not thrown away as it should be
8. to use something over again

Column II

a. air pollution
b. clinic
c. community
d. litter
e. pollute
f. recycle
g. sanitarian
h. water pollution

Reviewing Health Ideas

Number your paper from 1–8. Next to each number write the word that best completes the sentence. Choose the words from the list below.

air   harmful
clean   health
community   recycle
food   trash

1. Places to live, work, shop, and have fun can be found in a _____.
2. Sanitarians check to see if _____ is clean and safe to eat.
3. Gases from fuels burned in cars and trucks cause much _____ pollution.
4. At a water-treatment plant, _____ materials are taken out of water.
5. A _____ community is a healthy place to live, work, and play.
6. A community's garbage and _____ should be picked up often.
7. Litter can cause _____ problems in a community.
8. People help their community have less trash when they _____ things.

Understanding Health Ideas

Number your paper from 9–15. Next to each number write the word or words that best answer the question.

9. Who works to help keep people in a community healthy?
10. What can germs in food cause?
11. How can food workers keep from spreading harmful germs to the food they handle?
12. What can the health department do about air pollution in a community?
13. What might a sign next to polluted water say?
14. How do sanitation workers help keep a community clean and safe?
15. Where should litter be placed?

Thinking Critically

Write the answers on your paper. Use complete sentences.

1. What other ways can people in a community enjoy water that is safe for swimming?
2. What could you do around the outside of your home to help your community?

Using Metric

Metric Measures   ## Customary Measures

LENGTH

10 millimeters (mm) = 1 centimeter (cm)
100 centimeters = 1 meter (m)
1000 meters = 1 kilometer (km)

12 inches (in.) = 1 foot (ft.)
3 feet = 1 yard (yd.)
5280 feet = 1 mile (mi.)

MASS (WEIGHT)

1000 milligrams (mg) = 1 gram (g)
1000 grams = 1 kilogram (kg)
1000 kilograms = 1 metric ton (t)

16 ounces (oz.) = 1 pound (lb.)
2000 pounds = 1 ton (t.)

VOLUME

1000 milliliters (mL) = 1 liter (l)
1000 liters = 1 kiloliter (kl)

8 fluid ounces (fl. oz.) = 1 cup (c.)
2 cups = 1 pint (pt.)
2 pints = 1 quart (qt.)
4 quarts = 1 gallon (gal.)

TEMPERATURE

CELSIUS   FAHRENHEIT

Water boils 100° — 212° Water boils

Body temperature 37° — 98.6° Body temperature

Water freezes 0° — 32° Water freezes

Independent Study Guide

Use the *Independent Study Guide* to review
the lessons in each chapter. After you read
each lesson, answer the questions to find
out what you remember. Answering the
questions will help you learn the important
ideas in each lesson. You can also use the
study guide to help you review for the
chapter test.

Chapter 1 Study Guide

On a separate sheet of paper, write the word or words that best complete the sentence or answer the question.

Lesson 1

pages 18-19

1. Happiness, sadness, anger, worry, and surprise are _____.
2. What might a person's face show who feels happy?
3. Listening to a person's _____ is one way to tell how he or she feels.
4. People can show their feelings in the way they _____ or move.

Lesson 2

pages 20-21

1. A person might have scared feelings when he or she starts to learn _____ things.
2. What kind of feelings might a person have who is afraid of not doing something well?
3. Sometimes talking about scared feelings helps a person feel _____.
4. Who might a scared person talk with to feel less scared?

Lesson 3

pages 22-23

1. A _____ might give advice on how to change hurt feelings.
2. How can saying the words "I'm sorry" help when a person has hurt someone else's feelings?
3. A person who often does unkind things to others must act _____ to keep from hurting others' feelings.

Lesson 4
pages 24-25

1. Who might a sad person talk with to help himself or herself feel better?
2. Family members often know that a person whose pet has died feels very ▨▨▨.
3. Family members might suggest ▨▨▨ to help a sad person feel better.
4. Going ahead and crying often helps a sad person feel ▨▨▨.

Lesson 5
pages 26-27

1. A person might feel ▨▨▨ when things go wrong.
2. What active things might a child who feels angry do outside to feel better?
3. An angry person might do something for ▨▨▨ to help himself or herself feel better.
4. Who might an angry child ask for some work to do to help himself or herself feel better?

Lesson 6
pages 30-33

1. Too much arguing can ▨▨▨ people.
2. What can help people get along better with others and argue less?
3. A person who shows ▨▨▨ does his or her best to work with other people.
4. What can family members do around the home to show cooperation?
5. What are children showing toward a newcomer when they ask him or her to join their game?
6. A person shows ▨▨▨ when he or she tries to think of how another person feels?
7. What might a person say to someone who has made a mistake to show understanding?

Chapter 2 Study Guide

On a separate sheet of paper, write the word or words that best complete the sentence or answer the question.

Lesson
1
pages
40-43

1. What plan can be used to help choose healthy foods?
2. The four food group plan tells the number of daily _____ needed from each food group.
3. What are three ways that nutrients help the body?
4. The _____ in different foods work together to help the body stay healthy.

Lesson
2
pages
44-47

1. What kinds of foods make up a healthy meal?
2. Two servings are needed each day from the _____ group.
3. Three servings are needed each day from the _____ group.
4. Four servings are needed each day from both the bread-cereal and the _____ group.

Lesson
3
pages
48-49

1. A person needs to eat _____ kinds of vegetables.
2. Different kinds of vegetables give the body different kinds of _____.
3. The _____ needs the different kinds of nutrients in vegetables to stay healthy.
4. What ways other than fresh can vegetables be bought?

Lesson 4

pages 52-54

1. Healthy snacks should not be too ▧ or salty.
2. Sweet snacks can stick to the ▧ and harm them.
3. What are three healthy drinks?
4. Many foods eaten at meals contain salt so ▧ salt should not be added to the foods.
5. Milk, cheese, and yogurt are healthy snacks from the ▧ group.
6. What are some healthy snacks from the vegetable-fruit group?

Lesson 5

pages 56-57

1. A person needs to read the labels on cans to be a ▧ food shopper.
2. A wise food shopper can find out which kind of food will cost the least by looking at ▧.
3. What should a wise food shopper be willing to try?
4. The best tasting foods do not always ▧ the most.

Lesson 6

pages 60-61

1. What should you wash your hands with before handling foods?
2. What is removed from hands when they are washed?
3. What is removed from fresh fruits and vegetables when they are washed?
4. Some leftover foods should be put in a ▧.
5. Germs can grow in certain foods that get ▧.
6. Germs do not grow as quickly in ▧ places as they do in warm.

Chapter 3 Study Guide

On a separate sheet of paper, write the word or words that best complete the sentence or answer the question.

Lesson
1

pages
68-69

1. Bones, _____, nerves, and blood make up the inside of the body.
2. The smallest living parts of the body are _____.
3. Each kind of cell does a _____ job.
4. Cells of the same kind that are grouped together make up _____.
5. What kind of tissue do many bone cells together make up?

Lesson
2

pages
70-72

1. What are the muscles in the body attached to?
2. The muscles in the body work in _____.
3. Under the muscles in the body are _____.
4. What makes up a body's skeleton?
5. What body parts help a person move about?
6. What joint lets a person swing a bat?

Lesson
3

pages
74-75

1. The brain is an _____ made up of different kinds of tissues.
2. A person's _____ sends messages to the muscles about how to move.
3. Nerves are not all the _____ size.
4. Where are nerves found in the body?
5. The five senses are sight, _____, taste, hearing, and touch.

Lesson 4

pages 76-77

1. About how many times a minute does a child's heart beat?
2. What kind of tissue makes up most of the heart?
3. Blood carries oxygen and _____ to body cells.
4. What gas do body cells need to stay alive?
5. Blood picks up carbon dioxide and other _____ from body cells.
6. Blood travels to all parts of the body through little tubes called _____ vessels.

Lesson 5

pages 78-79

1. Where are the lungs found in the body?
2. Where does air breathed into the body through the nose or mouth go?
3. The heart pumps blood to the _____ where the blood picks up oxygen for body cells.
4. What gas is breathed out of the body?

Lesson 6

pages 80-83

1. When the body _____ food, it changes the form of the food.
2. Food is mixed with saliva so it can be _____.
3. What helps move food along the food tube?
4. Nutrients enter the blood through blood vessels in the _____ intestine.
5. Wastes leave the body through the _____ intestine.

Lesson 7

pages 86-87

1. Cells _____ to form new cells.
2. Your body becomes _____ as it adds new cells.
3. Each person grows in a way that is _____ for him or her.
4. Exercise helps _____ grow larger and stronger.
5. How does sleep help the body?

Chapter 4 Study Guide

On a separate sheet of paper, write the word or words that best complete the sentence or answer the question.

Lesson 1

pages 94-96

1. The hard, white material that helps protect the crown is called ▦.
2. The ▦ of a tooth are under the gum.
3. The center of a tooth has ▦ and blood vessels.
4. What two things does blood carry to the teeth?
5. The blood carries ▦ away from the teeth.
6. The nerves in a tooth send messages from the tooth to the ▦.

Lesson 2

pages 98-101

1. How many primary teeth will a baby have by age three?
2. Primary teeth help ▦ a person's face.
3. What can help keep primary teeth from coming out too soon?
4. What kind of tooth replaces a lost primary tooth?
5. If a permanent tooth does not have enough room, it may grow in ▦.
6. What can hold a space open for a permanent tooth that will grow in later?

Lesson 3

pages 102-103

1. Plaque is a sticky covering of harmful ▦.
2. What are two places where plaque forms?
3. The germs in plaque use ▦ to make an acid that can harm teeth.
4. A hole in a tooth is called a ▦.
5. Plaque can hurt ▦ as well as teeth.

1. Brushing teeth helps prevent ____.
2. How many times a day should teeth be brushed?
3. Brushing helps remove ____ and bits of food from the teeth and gums.
4. What can remove bits of food from between the teeth and near the gum line?
5. Dental floss should be gently moved up and down the ____ of a tooth.
6. Eating foods from the four food groups each day will help keep teeth and ____ healthy.
7. Try not to eat too many ____, sticky foods.
8. Sugar can stick to ____ and cause cavities.
9. Who uses special tools to clean plaque off teeth?
10. Even if you brush and floss your teeth, some ____ might stay on the teeth and harden.
11. Plaque can cause ____ disease.

1. What might an advertisement tell about a product?
2. What special seal should a person look for on a tube of toothpaste?
3. The ADA puts its seal on toothpastes that help ____ cavities.
4. Use a toothbrush that is the right ____ for your mouth.
5. A toothbrush should be flat on the top with soft, ____ edges.
6. You might find ____ dental floss easier to use if your teeth are close together.

Chapter 5 Study Guide

On a separate sheet of paper, write the word or words that best complete the sentence or answer the question.

Lesson 1

pages 121-123

1. What directions should you remember to look when crossing a street?
2. Each person is most responsible for his or her ▦ safety.
3. Following ▦ rules can help keep you safe.
4. Thinking of ways to ▦ an accident can help keep you safe.

Lesson 2

pages 124-125

1. Locked car doors prevent people from ▦ out of a car accidentally.
2. What should you wear when riding in a car?
3. Never bother the ▦ of a car.

Lesson 3

pages 126-127

1. An adult should help a child ▦ a bicycle to see if it is safe to drive.
2. Name four things needed on a bicycle to help keep a driver safe.
3. A bicycle driver should use ▦ signals when turning.

Lesson 4

pages 128-129

1. When unplugging a toaster, never pull on the ▦.
2. Never touch small electric appliances with ▦ hands.
3. What kinds of injuries can electricity cause?

Lesson 5

pages 130-131

1. Some cleaning products contain _____ that can be harmful.
2. Many products need to be used only in rooms with lots of _____ air.
3. What kinds of products should be stored away from food?

Lesson 6

pages 132-133

1. What should a swimmer do after reading a warning sign?
2. When should a swimmer call for help?
3. A swimmer should come out of the water if he or she feels _____ or cold.

Lesson 7

pages 136-139

1. What can be put in a home to warn of fire?
2. What can help keep a person from breathing in gases and smoke from a fire?
3. What should a person do if his or her clothes catch on fire?
4. Once a person gets out of a _____ home, he or she should not go back in for any reason.
5. A person whose home is on fire should _____ the fire department from a neighbor's home.

Lesson 8

pages 140-144

1. Try to get _____ help if someone is injured.
2. Who will help a person if he or she dials the number 0 on a telephone?
3. Listen to any _____ that are given when telephoning for help.
4. What should a small cut be washed with?
5. Press _____ on the bandage over a small cut if it keeps bleeding.
6. Run _____ water over an insect bite.

Chapter 6 Study Guide

On a separate sheet of paper, write the word or words that best complete the sentence or answer the question.

Lesson
1
pages
150-153

1. Medicines are a kind of _____.
2. Drugs can change how a person thinks, _____, or acts.
3. What kind of medicine do people need a doctor's order to buy?
4. Who fills the order for a prescription medicine?
5. What can be found on the label of a prescription medicine?
6. People do not need a prescription to buy _____ medicines.

Lesson
2
pages
154-157

1. Some medicines help cure diseases by killing _____ that cause the diseases.
2. What are some places where germs can be found?
3. Germs must get _____ the body to cause disease.
4. Germs can get into the _____ when a person breathes.
5. When germs upset the way the body works, a person becomes _____.
6. _____ cause strep throat and tuberculosis.
7. _____ called viruses can cause measles, mumps, and polio.
8. Virusus are much _____ than bacteria.
9. _____ is a disease caused by a virus that is very hard to get.

Lesson 3

pages
158-159

1. Medicines can _____ people if used the wrong way.
2. Prescription medicines should never be _____ with someone else.
3. An upset stomach or a headache could be a _____ effect from a medicine.
4. Where should medicines be stored to keep them away from small children?
5. Leave the _____ on all medicines so people can read them.
6. Most small children cannot open medicines with _____ caps.

Lesson 4

pages
160-161

1. What might a person do to help make a headache feel better other than taking medicine?
2. A person does not need to take _____ for every tiny ache or pain.
3. When you are upset, _____ might help you feel better.
4. Who should help a child decide if he or she needs a medicine to feel better?

Lesson 5

pages
164-167

1. Drinks that contain certain _____ are not healthy.
2. What are four drinks that contain caffeine?
3. What affect does caffeine have on the heart?
4. Too much caffeine causes some people to feel nervous or to lose _____.
5. Alcohol changes the way a person's _____ works.
6. The nicotine in a cigarette makes it _____ for a smoker to stop smoking.
7. What drug in cigarettes can cause heart disease?
8. What kind of warning is found on a cigarette package?

Chapter 7 Study Guide

On a separate sheet of paper, write the word or words that best complete the sentence or answer the question.

Lesson 1

pages 174-175

1. Physical fitness can help a person have more ____ playing games.
2. What can help a person work or play without getting tired easily?
3. Being physically fit can help you ____ your best.
4. A physically fit person has strong back, arm, ____, and stomach muscles.
5. Strong muscles help a person have good ____.
6. What can a person do comfortably if he or she has good posture?
7. Being physically fit might help prevent a child from having ____ diseases later in life.

Lesson 2

pages 176-177

1. People need ____ to move quickly and easily.
2. Agility is a part of physical ____.
3. What is a job that a person needs agility to do well?
4. Practicing certain stunts can help a person ____ his or her agility.

Lesson 3

pages 180-181

1. Try to ____ several times a day to stay healthy.
2. Walking to school can be good exercise if you walk ____.
3. At recess play ____ games to get exercise.
4. What are two exercises that a child might do after school?
5. Exercise at least fifteen to ____ minutes at a time.
6. You might need to ____ during exercise.

Lesson 4

pages 182-185

1. What happens to muscles in the body if they are not used?
2. Exercising helps make muscles ___.
3. Body muscles are made up of many muscle ___.
4. Muscle cells get ___ when a person exercises.
5. What is a good stretching exercise?
6. Muscles that stretch easily let you ___ and move easily.
7. What can a person do to help his or her heart work better?
8. The heart beats ___ during exercise.
9. Exercises that strengthen the heart also help the ___ work better.
10. What activities can you do to help your heart and lungs work better?

Lesson 5

pages 186-187

1. A good exercise plan should have exercises to make ___ strong.
2. A good exercise plan should have exercises to make the ___ and lungs work better.
3. Why should muscles be warmed up before exercising?
4. When should a person cool down his or her muscles?
5. A good way to warm up or cool down is by ___ your muscles.
6. Choose a ___ place to exercise.
7. Who should show a child the right way to do an exercise?
8. An exercise can be ___ if not done correctly.
9. Wear exercise clothes that let you move ___.

Chapter 8 Study Guide

On a separate sheet of paper, write the word or words that best complete the sentence or answer the question.

Lesson
1

pages
200-201

1. What has places for people to live, work, shop, and have fun?
2. Doctors, _____, nurses, and hospital workers help people stay healthy.
3. Many communities have a _____ department.
4. Workers in a health department help protect people from _____.
5. People can get health care at a _____.

Lesson
2

pages
202-205

1. What are four places where sanitarians check to see if food is clean and safe to eat?
2. What might the health department do about a place that does not have clean and safe food?
3. People might get _____ if they eat food with harmful germs.
4. What might workers with unclean hands spread to the food they handle?
5. Store some foods at _____ temperatures to help keep germs from growing quickly in them.
6. Storing food safely keeps _____ from growing.

Lesson
3

pages
206-207

1. People can get _____ from air pollution.
2. Who can help a community make plans to stop air pollution?
3. Most air pollution comes from _____.
4. Smoke and harmful gases _____ the air.

Lesson 4

pages 208-209

1. Drinking ___ water can make people sick.
2. Most communities have a ___ plant to make water safe to drink.
3. Water from a river or lake goes through ___ to a water-treatment plant.
4. Who tests water from a water-treatment plant to see if it is safe to drink?
5. What is water pollution?

Lesson 5

pages 210-211

1. What two things are picked up often to help keep a community clean?
2. Garbage will look and ___ terrible if it is not collected often.
3. Rats and ___ can spread harmful germs.
4. Sanitation workers collect garbage and trash in ___.

Lesson 6

pages 214-215

1. Do not leave ___ lying around your community.
2. Litter can make a community ___ and unattractive.
3. Litter can cause ___ problems.
4. Throw away litter in a ___ can or in a plastic bag.
5. There will be ___ trash to get rid of if you use things over again.
6. When you use things like paperbags over again, you ___ them.
7. Recycling helps make a ___ and safer community.
8. What are some objects that you might collect and bring to a recycling center?

Skills for Life Handbook

Use the activities in this handbook to learn and practice skills for life. These are skills that will help you deal with events in your life in good, healthful ways. Read stories about how people your age deal with some difficult situations. Then answer the questions about what these people have done or should do.

Deciding What to Do   You will learn how to judge choices to make wise and healthy decisions.

Judging Ads and Choosing the Best Product   You will learn how to use ads and labels to judge products in order to choose the healthiest ones.

Feeling Good About Yourself   You will learn how people can think good thoughts about themselves.

Learning How to Say No   You will learn when it is important to say no to avoid doing things that may be harmful or wrong. You will learn ways to say no.

NO FISHING POLLUTED

Dealing with Problems You will learn to deal with problems and feelings such as sadness and anger.

Setting Goals You will learn how to set healthy goals and then how to achieve them.

Getting Along with Others and Communicating Well You will learn ways to get along better with others. You will also learn ways to settle disagreements and communicate better.

Deciding What to Do

Jordan and his little sister Amy were playing catch in their backyard. After a while, their neighbor Tommy came over. Tommy asked Jordan to play football with him and some other boys. Jordan knew he was supposed to watch his sister. But he thought football would be more fun.

Jordan had a decision to make. It helps to think about the choices when making a decision. It also helps to think about the good and bad things that could happen from making each choice.

On a separate sheet of paper, answer these questions about Jordan's choices.

1. What are Jordan's choices?
2. What might be the good and bad things that could happen from making each choice?
3. Which choice do you think Jordan's parents would approve of? Why?
4. What do you think Jordan's decision should be? Why?

Dealing with Problems

Elena's mother started a new job last week. She works until 5:00 every day. She is not there when Elena gets home from school. Elena knows that her neighbors are home in the afternoons. She also knows she can call her mother at work if she needs something. However, Elena feels scared to be home alone after school. Elena does not want to worry her mother, but she feels like she needs help. Elena decides to talk to her teacher about her problem.

Answer the following questions on a sheet of paper.

1. What did Elena do to help with her problem?
2. Why was talking to her teacher the right thing to do?
3. What else could Elena do to help herself feel better?

Feeling Good About Yourself

Marty was invited to his cousin Frank's birthday party. Frank lives in another part of the city. Marty does not know most of his cousin's friends. Marty feels shy when he is around people he does not know. He does not want to go to the party.

"Let's go, Marty. It's time to leave," his mother says.

"Do I really have to go to Frank's party?" he asks.

"What's the matter? Why don't you want to go to the party?" asks his mother.

"I don't know Frank's friends. I'm going to feel dumb just sitting there," he says.

Pretend you are Marty's mother. What could you say to Marty to help him feel better about himself? Write two answers on a sheet of paper.

Getting Along with Others

Martha is watching TV alone in her living room. She is enjoying herself very much because her favorite show is on. Just before the end of the TV program, her brother Jake comes in the room and turns the channel. Martha becomes very angry and starts yelling at Jake. Their mother comes into the room a few minutes later. They are both screaming.

"I can't stand it when you scream at each other like this," their mother says. "You have to learn to get along with each other better."

Answer these questions on a separate sheet of paper.

1. What is one thing Jake could have done to get along better with Martha?
2. What is one thing Martha could have done to get along better with Jake?

Deciding What to Do

It is 3:00 and Emily is riding in the bus on her way home from school. She feels hungry. She begins thinking about what kind of snack she will have when she gets home.

When Emily arrives at her house, she heads straight for the kitchen. She sees bananas and apples on the table. She looks in the cupboard and finds cookies. Emily thinks about what she has been learning about healthy snacks in school. She loves cookies, but she knows that fruit would be a healthier snack.

Help Emily decide what to do. Answer the following questions on a sheet of paper.
1. What are Emily's choices?
2. Which choice would be the healthiest? How do you know?
3. What do you think Emily's decision should be? Why?

Choosing the Best Product

Charlie is at the supermarket with his mother. They are looking at cereals. Charlie's mother says that he can pick out a brand to buy for the family.

Charlie thinks about what he learned in school about healthy foods. He learned that nutrients in foods keep people healthy. He also learned that foods with too much sugar or salt are not very healthy.

Charlie's three favorite cereals are the ones in the pictures below. Even though he likes them all, Charlie thinks he should pick the cereal that is the healthiest.

On a separate sheet of paper, write which cereal you think Charlie should buy. Then write a sentence explaining your answer.

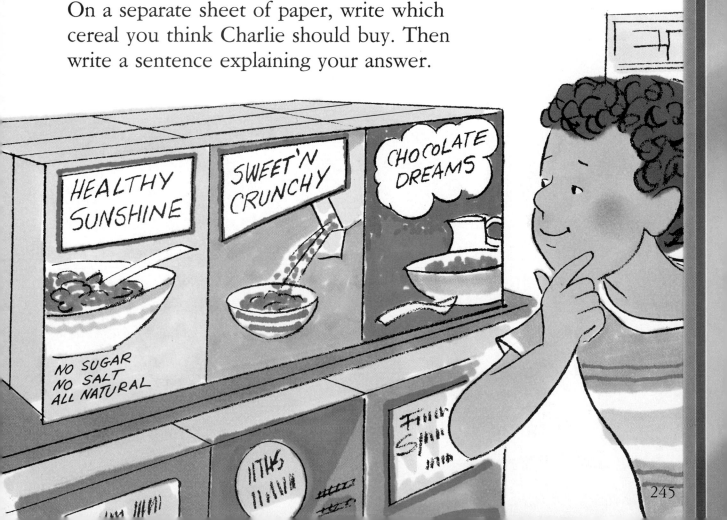

Setting Goals

A goal is something a person wants to do or achieve. A good goal is not too hard or too easy to reach. A goal should also be easy enough for the person to tell if it has been reached. For example, Joey made a goal of eating more vegetables. Then he realized it would be hard to tell when his goal would been reached. Joey changed his goal. He made a goal of eating vegetables every day. Now Joey will know each day if he has reached his goal.

Choose a nutrition goal for yourself. Write your goal on a separate sheet of paper. Then write how you will know if you have reached it.

LETTUCE   SQUASH   BROCCOLI

CARROTS   POTATOES   ASPARAGUS

Deciding What to Do

SKILLS FOR LIFE

Jennifer is walking to the movie theater with her classmate Kayla. Kayla has a problem with her joints. She is not able to move as easily as other people. Kayla uses braces to help her walk.

Suddenly, a boy runs by. He says they will miss the start of the movie unless they hurry. Jennifer thinks that maybe she should run ahead and get the tickets. But she does not want to leave Kayla alone.

Answer these questions about Jennifer's choices on another sheet of paper.

1. What would be the good and bad things that could happen from running ahead?
2. What would be the good and bad things that could happen from staying with Kayla?
3. Which choice do you think Jennifer should make? Why?

Dealing with Problems

Mitch broke his foot last week when he tripped over a rock. Now he has a cast on his leg. Mitch cannot do sports activities until his foot is healed. This might take another month.

Mitch is upset because he cannot play outside after school with his friends. He feels sad and lonely because he cannot do the activities that he enjoys.

Mitch learned in school how to deal with problems. He learned to do something you enjoy when things go wrong.

On another sheet of paper, write three things Mitch could do to help him deal with his problem.

Communicating Well

SKILLS FOR LIFE

When people smile or wave, they are using body language. Body language is the language that your body speaks by movements instead of words. Body language is the language you can see. The ways that people stand, sit, or hold their arms also make up body language. Understanding body language can help you learn how people are feeling.

The students in the picture below are reading reports about how the lungs work in front of their class. How do you think each person feels? How does body language help you understand how each person feels? Write your answers on a separate sheet of paper.

Feeling Good About Yourself

Willy is one of the smallest people in his class. Sometimes Willy feels upset because he is not growing as fast as others his age.

One day, Willy played basketball in the park with his friend Carlos. On the way home Carlos notices that Willy looks sad and asks him what is wrong. Willy tells Carlos that he does not like being so small. He says that it especially bothers him when they are playing basketball.

Pretend you are Carlos. On a separate sheet of paper, write three things you could say to Willy to help him feel better about his size.

Deciding What to Do

SKILLS FOR LIFE

Suzanna was biting into an apple. Suddenly she felt like she was crunching into a rock. Suzanna realized that a filling came out from one of her teeth.

Suzanna thought about what she should do. She knew that cavities should be filled to protect the teeth. However, Suzanna did not want to go back to her dentist. She remembered that it hurt when she got the cavity filled the first time.

Answer these questions about Suzanna's decision on another sheet of paper.

1. What would be the good and bad things that could happen if Suzanna did not get her cavity filled again?
2. What would be the good and bad things that could happen if Suzanna did have her cavity filled?
3. Which choice is more healthful?
4. Which choice do you think Suzanna's parents would want her to make?
5. What do you think Suzanna should do? Why?

Learning How to Say No

Lauren and her friend Kim were at the carnival together. They were having fun riding the ferris wheel, bumper cars, and roller coaster. Later they passed by the cotton candy stand.

"Oh boy, let's get some cotton candy!" Kim said.

"I don't know if it's such a good idea," said Lauren.

"Why not? What's the matter?" asked Kim.

"Cotton candy is bad for your teeth. Didn't you know that?" replied Lauren.

Lauren knew that sweet, sticky foods such as cotton candy are not good for teeth. She had two cavities the last time she was at the dentist's office. She did not want to have any cotton candy. She was afraid she would get more cavities.

On a separate sheet of paper, write three ways that Lauren could say no to Kim in a nice way.

Judging Ads

Ads can help people learn many things about health products. Ads can tell you how the product helps keep you healthy. Ads can tell you how to use the product. Ads can help you compare one product to another.

Sometimes ads do not include all the important health information that people want to know. This makes it harder for people to buy products.

The ads below are trying to sell toothpaste. On another sheet of paper, write one thing that could be added to each ad. Explain why this would help someone who wants to buy the best toothpaste.

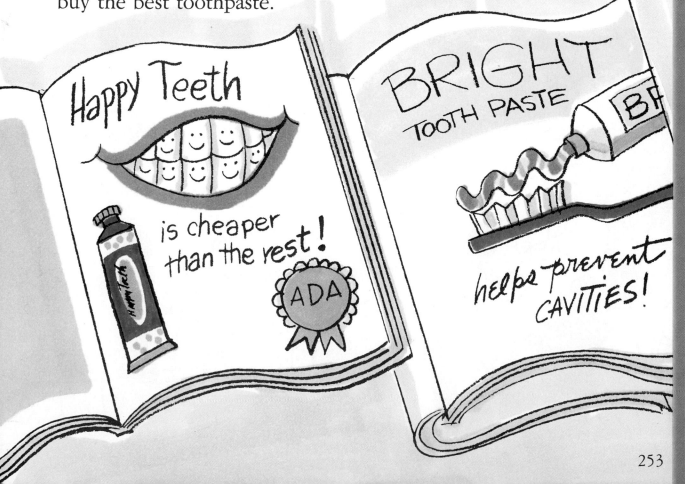

Happy Teeth is cheaper than the rest! ADA

BRIGHT TOOTH PASTE helps prevent CAVITIES!

Setting Goals

Lana has learned about brushing and flossing in school. She knows that brushing and flossing can help keep teeth and gums healthy. Lana brushes her teeth two times a day. However, she often forgets to floss her teeth.

Lana decides to set a goal of flossing her teeth four times per week. Her mother suggests that she make a plan to help her reach her goal. Lana puts a gold star on her plan each day that she remembers to floss her teeth. Lana is proud of herself for reaching her goal nearly every week.

How does making a plan help Lana reach her goal? Answer this question on a separate sheet of paper.

Deciding What to Do

Gina is at her friend Caroline's house. It is a beautiful day and they want to go bike riding. Gina does not have her bike with her. Caroline says that Gina can borrow her sister's bike.

The girls walk into the garage to get the bikes. Caroline pulls out her bike. Then she points to her sister's bike. Gina can see that the bike is too big for her. Gina wants to go bike riding, but she thinks it may not be safe for her to ride this bike.

Answer these questions on a separate sheet of paper.
1. What are Gina's choices?
2. Which choice would be the safest?
3. What do you think Gina's decision should be? Why?

Learning How to Say No

Evan and his neighbor Chris are swimming in the pool at the park. They are swimming in the shallow end of the pool. After a while, Chris suggests that they swim down to the deep end.

Evan does not think that he and Chris are good enough swimmers to go into the deep end. He thinks Chris wants to go to the deep end to show off. Evan does not want to swim in the deep end. However, he does not want Chris to think that he is a baby.

On a separate sheet of paper, write three ways Evan could say no to Chris.

Feeling Good About Yourself

Eddie took his four-year-old cousin Max for a walk around the neighborhood. They walked several blocks. Eddie made sure they walked on the sidewalk and stopped at all corners. He told Max to look both ways before crossing the street. They had a safe and enjoyable walk together.

When Eddie returned from the walk, he felt proud of himself for following all the safety rules on his walk with Max. He wanted to tell his parents about it.

On a separate sheet of paper, write three things Eddie could tell his parents that show he feels good about himself for being safe.

Communicating Well

Everyone in the Johnson family wears their safety belts in the car. They all know that safety belts help protect people from injury if an accident happens.

One day, Mrs. Johnson was taking her daughter Crystal to the mall. Crystal's friend Melanie was coming too. Crystal and Mrs. Johnson put on their safety belts right away.

"Don't forget to put on your safety belt," Crystal said to Melanie.

Melanie said, "Oh, I don't wear those."

Finish this conversation on a separate sheet of paper. Have Crystal and Mrs. Johnson explain to Melanie why she should always wear a safety belt in a car.

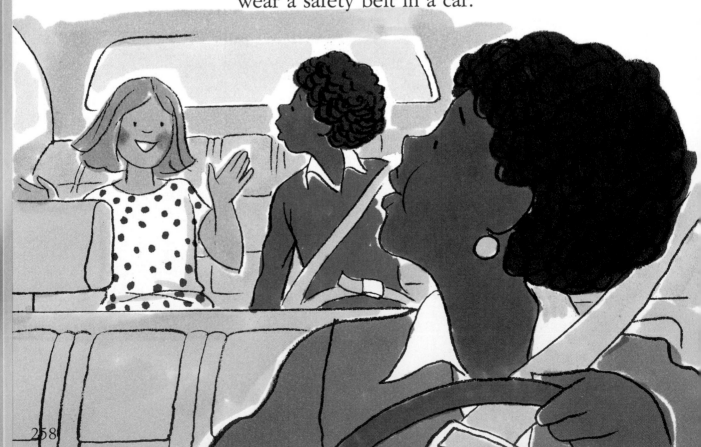

Deciding What to Do

Robin is at her friend Gayle's house for the afternoon. Robin and Gayle are in the basement. Gayle's parents are outside.

"Hey, I found some cigarettes," Gayle says to Robin. "Want to try one?"

"Are you crazy?" responds Robin.

"What's the matter? My parents will never find out," says Gayle.

Robin knows that smoking cigarettes is unhealthy. She knows that people her age are not allowed to smoke. Robin also thinks about her parents. She knows they would be very upset if they knew she smoked. Robin decides not to smoke.

Answer these questions on a sheet of paper.
1. Why is Robin's decision the right decision?
2. What does Robin know that helps her make her decision?

Communicating Well

Belinda is home with her older brother Kevin. Belinda comes downstairs and tells Kevin that she does not feel very well. Kevin suggests that she take some medicine.

Belinda has been learning about taking medicine in school. Belinda knows that medicine can harm people if used in the wrong way. She also learned that only an adult should give medicine to a child. Belinda does not think she should take any medicine from her brother.

Pretend you are Belinda. Write three things you could say to Kevin to explain why it is not safe to take medicine from him. Write your answers on a separate sheet of paper.

Learning How to Say No

Tony and his older cousin Rosanne are at a birthday party for their grandfather. Their grandfather is seventy-five years old. Many people are at Tony's house celebrating this important birthday.

Rosanne comes up to Tony and says, "Let's go get Aunt Mona's extra alcohol."

"We can't. We're too young." Tony says.

"Why not?" replies his sister. "Everyone is so busy. They will never notice. Don't you even want to try it?"

Tony does not want any alcohol. He knows that alcohol is a drug that affects the brain. He knows it can be harmful.

On another sheet of paper, write two different ways that Tony could say no to Rosanne.

Dealing With Problems

Simon is having a bad day. He tripped on the way to school and tore a hole in his pants. He did not do well on his math quiz. After school, his mother yelled at him because he forgot to feed the cat. Now he is having problems with his science homework.

Simon does not feel very well. He has a stomach ache and his head hurts a little. He wonders if he should take some medicine.

Answer these questions on a separate sheet of paper.
1. Why might Simon not be feeling well?
2. What things can Simon do instead of taking medicine to help him feel better?

Deciding What to Do

SKILLS FOR LIFE

Leslie knows that getting enough exercise every day helps keep people healthy. After school, Leslie likes to go outside to play with her neighbors.

Leslie walks outside and sees her friends Dina and Kathy sitting in the sun. They invite her join them. In the other direction she sees other people she knows playing kickball. Leslie thinks about what she should do.

Answer these questions about Leslie's decision on a separate sheet of paper.

1. What are Leslie's choices?
2. Which choice would be the most healthy?
3. What would be good and bad things that could happen from each choice?
4. What do you think Leslie should do? Why?

Setting Goals

Drew enjoys riding his bike. After seeing a bike race on TV, Drew gets an idea. He wants to work harder to develop more strength. Drew wants to ride faster and farther. Maybe he will even enter a bike race himself.

Drew sets a goal to ride around the bike path at the park in ten minutes. He can now ride around the park in fifteen minutes. He wants to reach his goal in one month.

On a separate sheet of paper, answer the following questions about Drew's goal.
1. Did Drew make a good goal for himself? How do you know?
2. What might Drew do to reach his goal?
3. How will Drew know if he has reached his goal?

Feeling Good About Yourself

Drew has worked hard to reach his goal. He can now ride around the bike path in the park in ten minutes. Drew has also become more physically fit.

Drew decides to enter a bike race for people his age. He thinks he can win the race because he now has more strength. Drew tries very hard, but he does not win the bike race. Drew tells his father that he feels awful because he lost.

"Drew, you should not feel bad," his father says. "You should feel proud of yourself because of how hard you worked. Just think about how much your strength has improved!"

On a sheet of paper, write three things Drew could say that show he is now thinking good things about himself.

Getting Along with Others

Connie and Janet both like to jump rope. They do this exercise at recess almost every day. They know jumping rope can help keep their heart and lungs healthy.

Cheryl is a new girl at school. Connie and Janet ask Cheryl to jump rope with them. Cheryl is not very good. She is not as agile as the other girls. Connie starts making fun of Cheryl because of this. Janet thinks Connie is being mean.

Pretend you are Janet. You want Connie to get along with Cheryl. What could you say to Connie that will help her become Cheryl's friend? Write your answer on another sheet of paper.

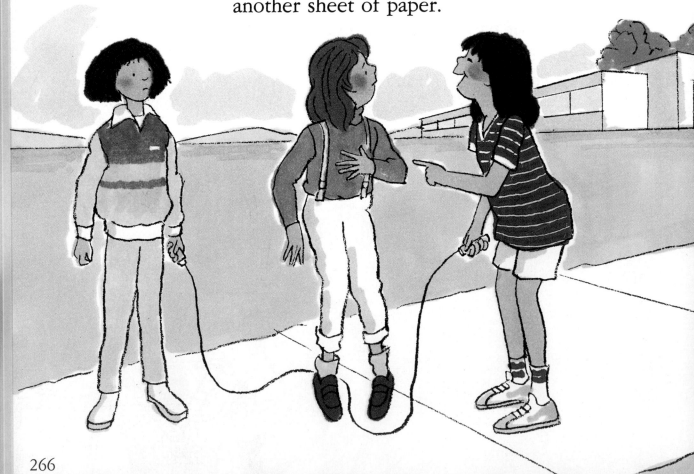

Deciding What to Do

Roger's community is having a paper drive. People in the community are collecting bundles of paper to recycle. Roger knows that recycling helps the community.

Roger told his mother that he would gather the extra papers in the house. Then he would help take them to the recycling center. However, he is now playing with his friend Jimmy and does not want to stop. Roger has to decide if he will help collect the papers or keep playing with his friend.

Answer these questions on a separate sheet of paper.

1. Which of Roger's choices is more healthful?
2. Which choice do you think Roger's parents would want him to make?
3. What decision do you think Roger should make? Why?

Learning How to Say No

Greg and Steve are on a camping trip with their Boy Scout group. They are walking along the edge of the lake near the campground. They see a sign that says, "No Fishing. Polluted."

Greg and Steve are disappointed. They have both been looking forward to fishing on this trip.

Greg suggests, "Why don't we try to take down the sign."

Steve says, "You and your crazy ideas. Just keep walking."

On a separate sheet of paper write two other ways Steve could have said no to Greg.

Setting Goals

Kelly knows that some parts of her community have litter. Kelly knows that litter can cause health problems. She wants to do something to help make her community cleaner and healtheir.

Kelly decides to set a goal to help reduce litter. Kelly remembers that a good goal is not too hard or too easy. She wants to be able to reach her goal.

Answer these questions on a separate sheet of paper.

1. What could be a goal Kelly could set to help reduce litter?
2. What things could Kelly do to help reach her goal?

Glossary

Glossary

Pronunciation Key

The pronunciation of each word is shown just after the word, in this way: **ab bre vi ate** (ə brē′vē āt). The letters and signs used are pronounced as in the words below. The mark ′ is placed after a syllable with primary or heavy accent, as in the example above. The mark ′ after a syllable shows a secondary or lighter accent, as in **ab bre vi a tion** (ə brē′vē ā′shən).

a	hat, cap	**j**	jam, enjoy	**u**	cup, butter
ā	age, face	**k**	kind, seek	**ù**	full, put
ä	father, far	**l**	land, coal	**ü**	rule, move
		m	me, am		
b	bad, rob	**n**	no, in	**v**	very, save
ch	child, much	**ng**	long, bring	**w**	will, woman
d	did, red			**y**	young, yet
		o	hot, rock	**z**	zero, breeze
e	let, best	**ō**	open, go	**zh**	measure, seizure
ē	equal, be	**ô**	order, all		
ėr	term, learn	**oi**	oil, voice	**ə**	represents:
		ou	house, out		**a** in about
f	fat, if				**e** in taken
g	go, bag	**p**	paper, cup		**i** in pencil
h	he, how	**r**	run, try		**o** in lemon
		s	say, yes		**u** in circus
i	it, pin	**sh**	she, rush		
ī	ice, five	**t**	tell, it		
		th	thin, both		
		ŦH	then, smooth		

A

accident (ak′sə dənt), unexpected event that could harm someone.

agility (ə jil′ə tē), the ability to move quickly and easily.

alcohol (al′kə hôl), a drug that can be harmful and is found in beer, wine, and liquor.

air pollution (pə lü′shən), materials in the air that are harmful to health when breathed in.

appliance (ə plī′əns), a machine used to do a certain job.

argue (är′gyü), give reasons for or against something.

argument (är′gyə mənt), discussion by persons who do not agree.

artist (är′tist), a person who paints pictures.

B

bacteria (bak tir′ē ə), certain living things made of one cell that can cause diseases such as strep throat and tuberculosis.

blood vessel (ves′əl), a tube through which blood travels in the body.

bread-cereal group, the food group that has grains and foods made from grains.

C

caffeine (kaf′ēn), a drug found in drinks such as coffee, tea, cola, and cocoa. Too much caffeine might harm the body.

carbon dioxide (kär′bən
dī ok′sīd), a colorless waste
gas given off by the cells.

cavity (kav′ə tē), a hole in a
tooth caused by acid.

cell (sel), the smallest living part
of the body.

clinic (klin′ik), a place where
people can get health care.

consideration
(kən sid′ə rā′shən), thinking
about another person's feelings.

cooperation (kō op′ə rā′shən),
working together with other
people.

crown (kroun), the part of a
tooth above the gum.

D

dental floss (den′tl flos), strong
thread that can help clean
between the teeth.

dental hygienist (hī jē′nist), a
person who helps a dentist and
cleans and X-rays teeth.

dietitian (dī′ə tish′ən), a person
who plans daily meals that
have the right number of
servings from each food group.

digest (də jest′), change food to
a form that the cells in the body
can use.

disease (də zēz′), an illness.

drug (drug), a substance used
to treat, prevent, or cure
disease.

E

electric shock, an injury caused
by electricity moving through
the body.

enamel (i nam′əl), the hard
outer covering that protects a
tooth.

F

feelings, the way a person feels about something.

first aid, immediate care given for an injury.

I-J

injury (in′jər ē), damage to the body.

joint (joint), a place where bones fit together; different joints allow different kinds of movement.

L

litter, trash that is not thrown away as it should be.

large intestine (in tes′tən), the organ of the body where wastes are passed out of the body.

M

meat-poultry-fish-bean group, the food group that has meats, poultry, fish, nuts, eggs, and beans.

milk-cheese group, the food group that has milk and foods made from milk.

N

nicotine (nik′ə tēn′), a drug in tobacco that can harm a smoker's heart.

nutrient (nü′trē ənt), a substance from food that is needed for health and growth.

O

organ (ôr′gən), a group of different tissues that work together to do the same job.

over-the-counter medicine, a medicine that can be bought without a prescription.

oxygen (ok′sə jən), a colorless gas cells take in to stay alive.

P

pasteurize (pas′chə rīz′), heat to a high enough temperature and for a long enough time to kill harmful germs.

permanent (pėr′mə nənt) **teeth**, the second set of teeth.

pharmacist (fär′mə sist), a person who fills a doctor's order for a prescription medicine.

pharmacy assistant (fär′mə sē ə sis′tənt), a person who helps a pharmacist fill orders for prescription medicines.

physical (fiz′ə kəl) **fitness**, the ability to exercise without getting tired or injured easily.

plaque (plak), a sticky material made up of germs.

poison (poi′zn), a substance that if taken into or put on the body can be dangerous to life or health.

pollute (pə lüt′), to make dirty.

posture (pos′chər), the way a person holds his or her body.

prescription (pri skrip′shən), a written direction or order for preparing and using a medicine.

prescription (pri skrip′shən) **medicine**, a medicine that can be bought only with a doctor's order.

primary (prī′mer′ē) **teeth**, first twenty teeth that come through a child's gums.

R

recycle (rē sī′kəl), to use something over again.

S-T

saliva (sə lī′və), a juice in the mouth that helps soften food.

sanitarian (san′ə ter′ē ən), a person who checks to see if food is clean and safe to eat.

sense, sight, hearing, smell, taste, or touch.

sharing, using something together.

side effect, an unwanted change caused by taking a medicine.

small intestine (in tes′tən), the organ of the body where nutrients in food enter the blood.

strength, being strong and able to do many different physical activities.

tissue (tish′ü), a group of cells that look alike.

U-V

understanding, knowing what another person is feeling.

vaccine (vak′sēn′), a medicine that can prevent a disease.

vegetable-fruit group, the food group that has vegetables and fruits.

virus (vī′rəs), a tiny germ that can cause diseases such as measles, mumps, and polio.

W-X

water pollution (pə lü′shən), materials in water that are harmful to health.

X-ray technologist (tek nol′ə jist), a person who uses an X-ray machine to take pictures of parts inside the body.

Index

Index

*A **bold-faced** number indicates a page with a picture about the topic.*

C

Caffeine, 164, 169
Calm, 140–141, 143
Carbon dioxide, 76, 79, 89
Careers, 29, 51, 85, 111, 135,
163, 179, 213
Carefulness, 123
Cavity, **102,** 103, 107,
108–109, 112, 117
Chemicals, 60
Chest, **78**
Children and exercise, 184, **185**
Cigarette health warning, **166**
Clinic, 201, 217
Clothes and fire safety, **137**
Community, **200–201**
  clean and safe, 210
  health, 200–215
  workers, 200–215
Consideration, **32–33,** 35
Cooperation, 30, 35
Crossing streets, **122–123**
Crown (tooth), **94,** 96, 117

D

Dental floss, **106, 115,** 117
Dental hygienist, **108, 111,**
114, 117

Dentist, 101, **108–109,** 113,
114, 200
Dietitian, **51**
Disease
  and nicotine, 166
  and medicine, 154–157
  community protection, 201
  prevention of, 174
Doctor, **150,** 200
  advice on medicine, 161
Drugs, 150, 167
Drugstore workers, **163**

E

Electric appliance safety,
128–129
Electric shock, 128, 145
Enamel, **94–95,** 117
Energy, 41
Enjoyment, 27
Exercise, 26, 35, **87**
  and strong muscles, **182,** 183
  health needs, **180–181,**
    184, **185**
  safety rules, **186–187**
  warm-up and cool-down, 186
Exercise program, **188–193**
Eyes, 75

F

G

H

Hair, 68
Harmful drugs, 166–167
Headache, 160
Health department workers, 201, 206–207, **208 209**
Health warnings, 166
Health workers, 200, 202, **203**
Healthy drinks, 52–54, **55, 164**
Healthy food, 40–62, 87
  choices, **40–41**
Healthy meals, **44–45, 46–47, 48–49**
Healthy snacks, **52–55**
Hearing, 75
Heart, **76**
  and exercise, 184, 186
  disease, 166
  disease prevention, 174
  pumping, **79**
Heartbeat, 76–77
  and caffeine, 164
Helping others, 27
Hospital workers, 200
Household products safety, **130–131**

I

Injury, 123, 140–143, 145
  fires, 136–139
  first aid, **141–142**
  safe treatment for, 140–143
Insect bite, first aid for, **143**
Intestines, **81–83**

J

Jawbone, 94–95
Joints, **72**
Julian, Percy, **168**

L

Labels
  food, **56–57**
  household products, **130–131**
  over-the-counter medicine, **152–153**
  prescription medicine, **150–151,** 153, 158, 163
Large intestine, 81, **82,** 83
Lifeguard, **132**
Litter, 214, **215,** 217
Lungs, **79**
  and exercise, 184, 186
  cancer, 166

M

Marijuana cigarettes, 166
Measles, **156**
Meat-poultry-fish-bean group,
  43, 44–45, 63
Medicine, 150–151, **152–153,**
  157
  help for disease, 154–155, 157
  safe use of, 158, **159,** 162
  sometimes unnecessary,
    160–161
Microscope, **68**
Milk-cheese group, **43,** 44–45, 63
Mistakes, 33
Mouth, **83**
Movement
  messages to muscles, 74
  muscles pulling bones, 70–72
Mumps, **156**
Muscles, 68–69
  and bones, **70, 71,** 72, 73
  and digestion, 80–81, 82
  cells, **69, 182**
  exercising of, 174, **182–183,**
    184, **185, 186–187**

N

Nails, 68
Nerves, 68–69, **74**

cells, **69**
Nicotine, 166, 167, 169
Nutrients, 40–41, 43, 48–49, 63
  for teeth, 94
  supplied to cells, 76, 81

O

Organs, 89
  brain, **74**
  digestive, **80–83**
  heart, **76–77**
  lungs, **78–79**
Others, 23, 35
Over-the-counter medicine,
  152–153, 160–161, 169
Oxygen, 76, 78–79, 94

P

Pain, 160–161
  and medicine, **158**
Pasteur, Louis, **62**
Permanent teeth, 98,
  100–101, 117
Pet death, 24–25
Pharmacist, 150, **151,** 152–153
Pharmacy assistant, **163**

W

Walking, 180–181, 184
  posture, 174
Washing
  fruits and vegetables, **60–61**
  hands, 60–61, 203
Water
  for safe drinking, 201
  for safe swimming, **209**
  pollution of, **208–209,** 217
  safety rules, **129, 132–133**
Water-treatment plant, **208–209**

X

X ray, **88**
X-ray technologist, **85**

Acknowledgments (Picture Credits)

Page 34: Ben Weaver/Camera 5
Page 62: Courtesy Parke-Davis, Division of
    Warner-Lambert Company
Pages 68, 69: Ed Reschke (all)
Page 88: Bettmann Archive
Page 102: Courtesy Naval Dental Research Institute
Pages 103, 105: Copyright by the American Dental
    Association. Reprinted by permission.
Page 116: Courtesy *M.D. Magazine,* October 1974
Page 154 (l): © 1985 Martin M. Rotker/Taurus
Page 155 (c): Michael Abbey/Photo Researchers
    (r): © 1984 Martin M. Rotker/Taurus
Page 156 (l, c): Centers for Disease Control, Atlanta,
    GA. 30333
    (r): Omicron/Photo Researchers Inc.
Page 157: Prof. Luc Montagnier/Institut Pasteur/
    CNRI/Science Photo Laboratory/
    Photo Res.
Page 168: Wide World Photos, Inc.
Page 182 (t): Ed Reschke
Page 194: Focus on Sports, Inc.

All photographs not credited are the property of Scott,
Foresman and Company. These include photographs
taken by the following photographer:

James L. Ballard: Pages 16–17, 18–19, 21, 22–23,
    24–25, 26–27, 28, 29, 31, 32–33, 35, 38–39, 40–41,
    42–43, 44–45, 48–49, 50, 51, 52–53, 54, 55, 58, 61,
    63, 66–67, 73, 75, 78, 79, 84, 85, 86–87, 89, 92–93,
    97, 106, 107, 108, 110, 111, 114, 115, 117,
    120–121, 122–123, 124, 125, 126–127, 128–129,
    132–133, 134, 135, 136, 137, 141, 142, 143, 145,
    148–149, 151, 159, 161, 162, 163, 164–165,
    167, 169, 172–173, 175, 176–177, 178, 179,
    180–181, 182–183, 185, 186–187, 188–189,
    190–191, 192–193, 195, 198–199, 203, 204–205,
    208–209, 210, 211, 212, 213, 215, 216, 217